WELL YOUR WORLD
YOUTUBE FAVORITES!
VOLUME 2!

REEBS & DILLON HOLMES

OUR FAVORITE PLANT-BASED RECIPES | SALT, OIL, & SUGAR FREE

*For WJH.
These books were his idea.*

YOUTUBE FAVORITES! - VOLUME 2

© Reebs & Dillon Holmes 2023

https://wellyourworld.com

All Rights Reserved. No part of this book may be used or reproduced in any manner whatsoever without written permission. You may print the pages of this digital book for personal use only.

Print Edition ISBN # 979-8-9860530-6-6
Digital Edition ISBN # 979-8-9860530-7-3

The ideas, concepts, recipes, and opinions expressed in this book are intended to be used for educational purposes only. Our books and recipes are sold with the understanding that author and publisher are not rendering medical advice of any kind, nor are the books or recipes intended to replace medical advice, nor to diagnose, prescribe or treat any disease, condition, illness, or injury.

It is imperative that before beginning any diet or exercise program, including any aspects of this book, you receive full medical clearance from a qualified physician.

Authors claim no responsibility to any person or entity for any liability, loss, or damage caused or alleged to be caused directly or indirectly as a result of the use, application, or interpretation of the material in this book.

WELL YOUR WORLD!

What a year it has been both at home and here at Well Your World. At the time of launching our first cookbooks last year we welcomed baby Luka into the world. Now I'm about to give birth to a second baby boy! It seems every time I am pregnant, I go to work producing cookbooks!

We've been so thrilled with the growth that Well Your World has experienced over the past year. Although our core message has always been about simplifying your healthy whole plant food diet, I feel like it took us until this year to really clarify the way we deliver that message. So many of us get into healthy eating thinking we need to be absolutely perfect by eating an extreme variety of health foods each and every day. In fact, the truth is that health comes more from what we remove from our diets than what we add.

There is no need to go nuts complicating your daily routine with tricks and hacks to extract every last molecule of nutrition from the food. When all you eat are whole plant foods including veggies, fruit, and starches, you'll get more than enough nutrients in your diet. You won't need to worry about protein or super foods or any stringent routine or technique. Just figure out the foods and flavors you love to eat day in day out, and repeat the simple, fast methods that get those foods into your belly.

If you shop and eat from a standard list of easy-to-find ingredients like the ones we use in all of our recipes, then you'll almost always have what you need to browse our cookbooks and whip something up in as little as 20 minutes. Add a bunch of "nutrient chasing" and complexity and you're sure to hit burnout very quickly. We always say that the simpler you make your food prep the more likely you are to stick to this way of eating forever.

Thank you for the kindness and support you have shown us. We truly love our jobs, especially when we get to interact with all of you on our live streams and cooking shows. Be on the lookout for lots more from Well Your World in the coming months and years!

xoxo, Reebs

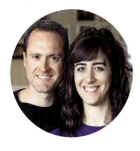

- 🌐 www.wellyourworld.com
- ▶ youtube.com/wellyourworld
- facebook.com/groups/wellyourworld
- @wellyourworld
- ✉ hello@wellyourworld.com

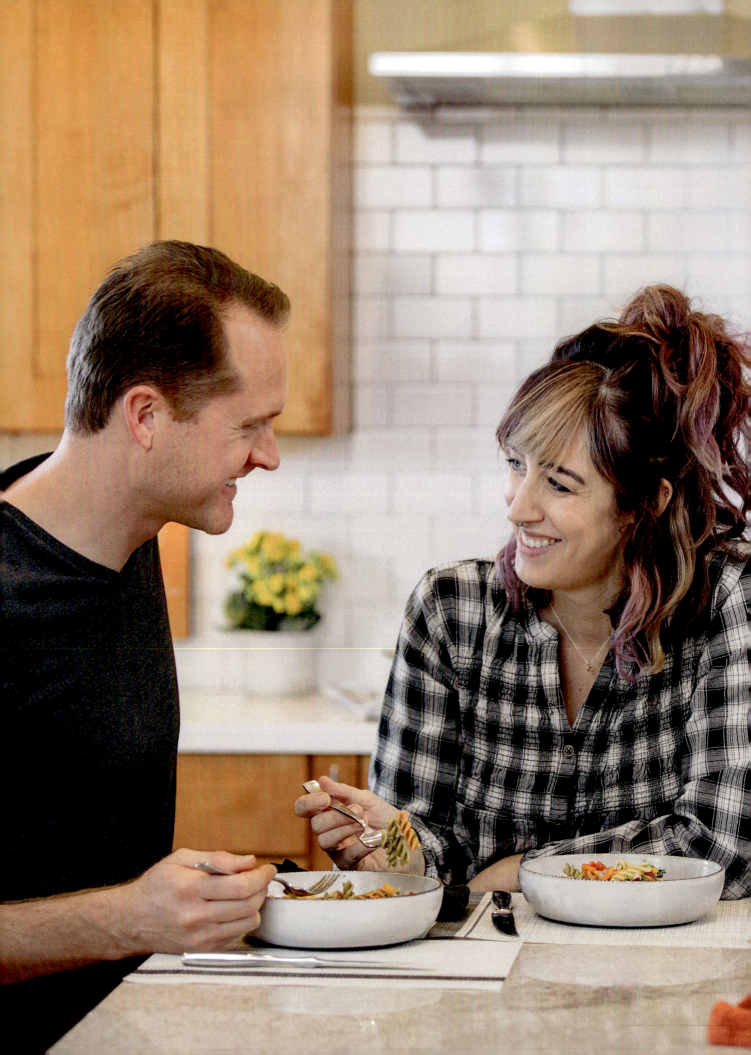

PLANT BASED DIET 101

For those of you who are new to this way of eating, let me go over what our diet includes and excludes. Check out the list below!

INCLUDES:

- Leafy greens
- Vegetables
- Starches - Potatoes, Legumes, Whole grains
- Fresh fruit
- Nuts, seeds, & avocado (whole fats)
- Plant-based milks

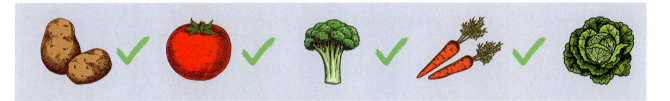

EXCLUDES:

- Animal products - meat, dairy, eggs, seafood
- Processed oils
- Heavily processed or extracted foods
- Refined sweeteners
- Bleached flours, white bread, white pasta

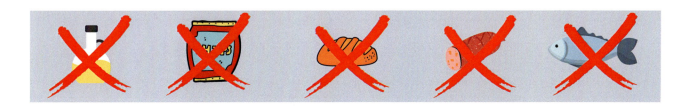

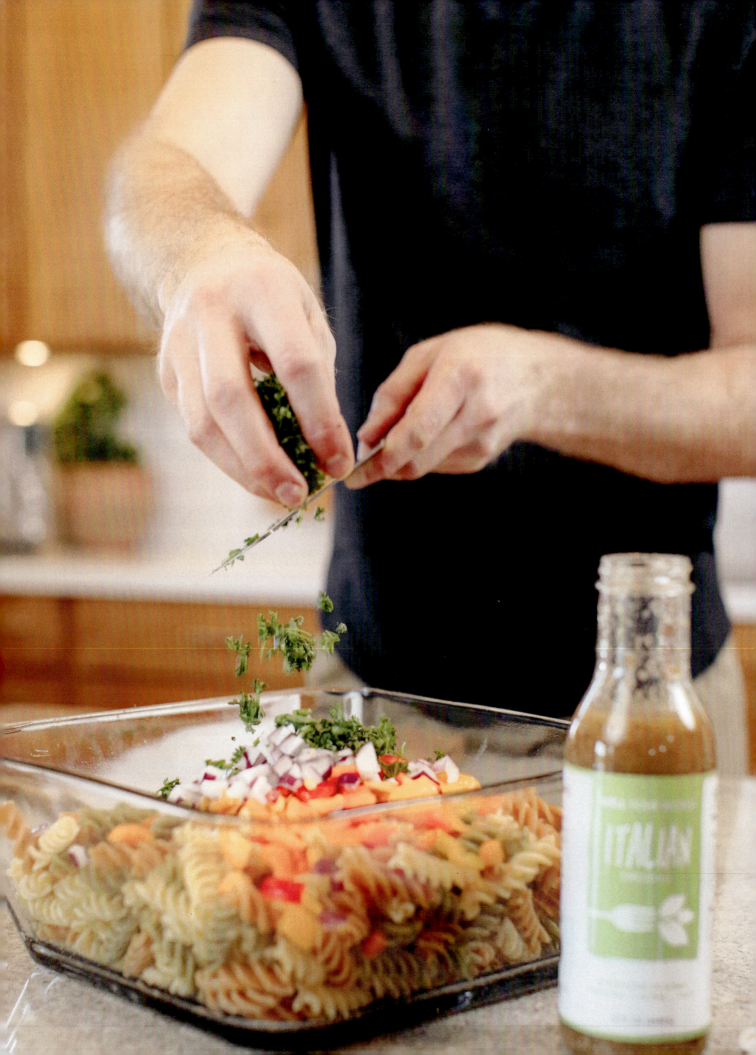

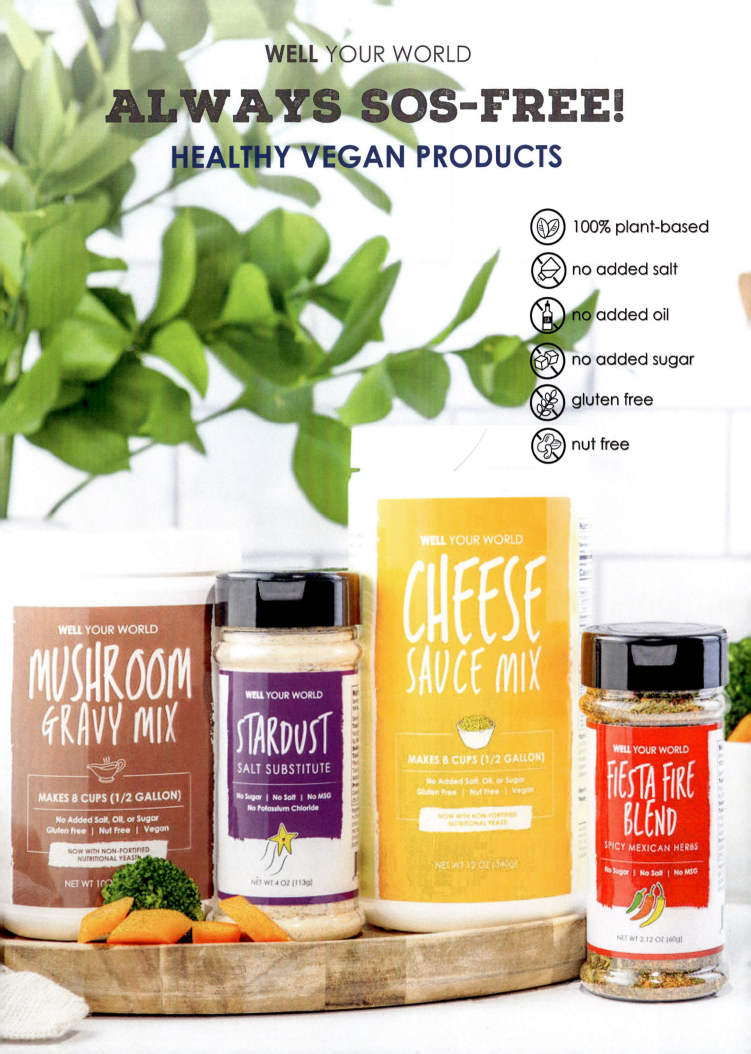

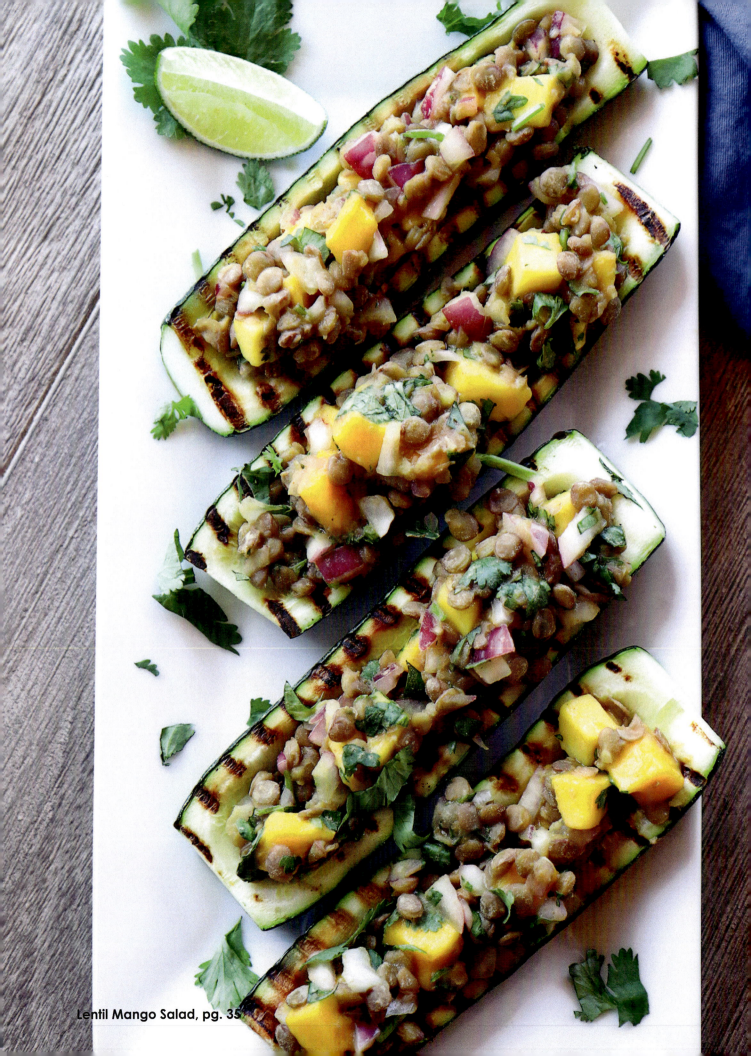

Lentil Mango Salad, pg. 35

WHY SOS-FREE?

All of the recipes on our YouTube channel, in our live cooking show, Well Your Weekend, as well as all of our food products are free of added salt, oil, and sugar.

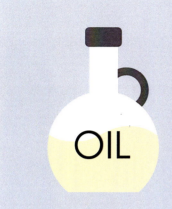

Oil is without question the worst offender in terms of calorie density. It is highly processed, void of any notable nutrient content, and 100% fat. Oil is 4,000 calories per pound! Plus, it is responsible for many adverse health problems such as obesity, heart disease, and type 2 diabetes.

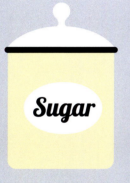

Sugar generally isn't as bad as oil in terms of detrimental health effects, but it is still very calorie dense, at 1,800 calories per pound. Higher calorie density = richer flavor = harder to stop eating. Before you know it, you've just eaten a bunch of useless calories.

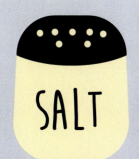

Salt is tricky because it doesn't have any calories. However, it can still hijack your taste buds and cause you to eat more than you otherwise would have. Many people avoid salt for other health reasons as well, i.e. hypertension.

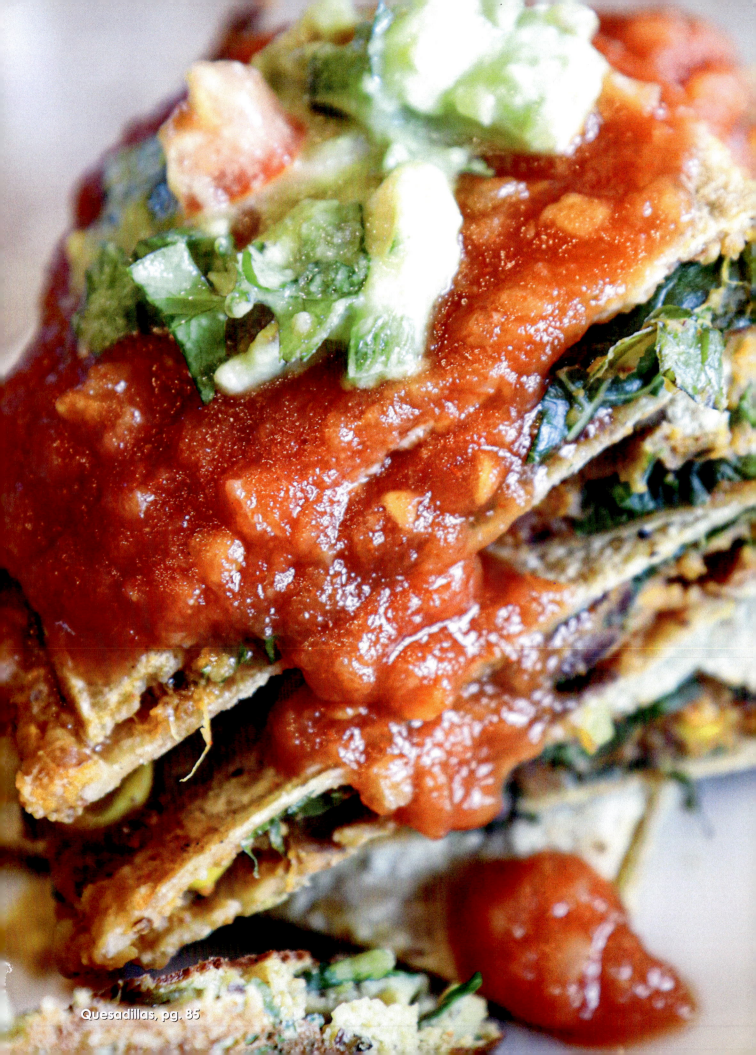

Quesadillas, pg. 85

WHAT IS CALORIE DENSITY?

Without getting too science-y, calorie density is just a way of explaining how many calories are in a given volume of food. For example, a pound of vegetables is roughly 100 calories, while a pound of processed oil contains 4,000 calories. That is quite a difference!

By centering your diet around foods with the lowest calorie density, you can lose the excess weight while staying full and satiated, all without the guilt.

I do include whole plant fats in my diet, such as nuts, seeds, and avocado, as well as in some of the recipes in this book. If you are looking for steady weight loss or are following a truly low fat diet, feel free to make modifications in order to omit or reduce these items.

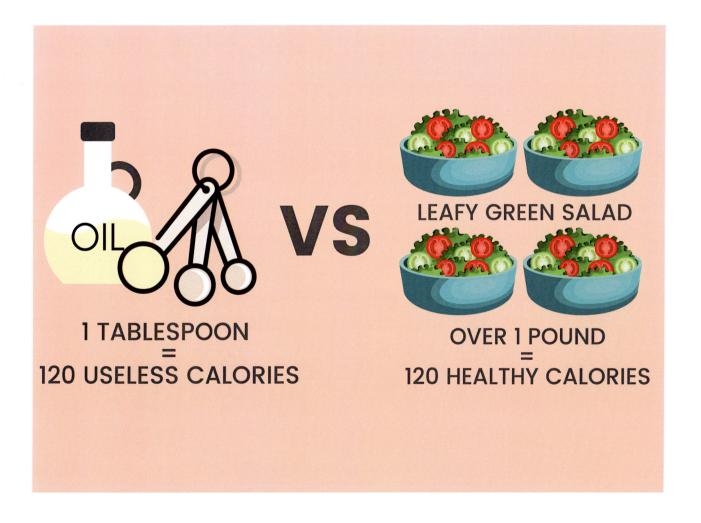

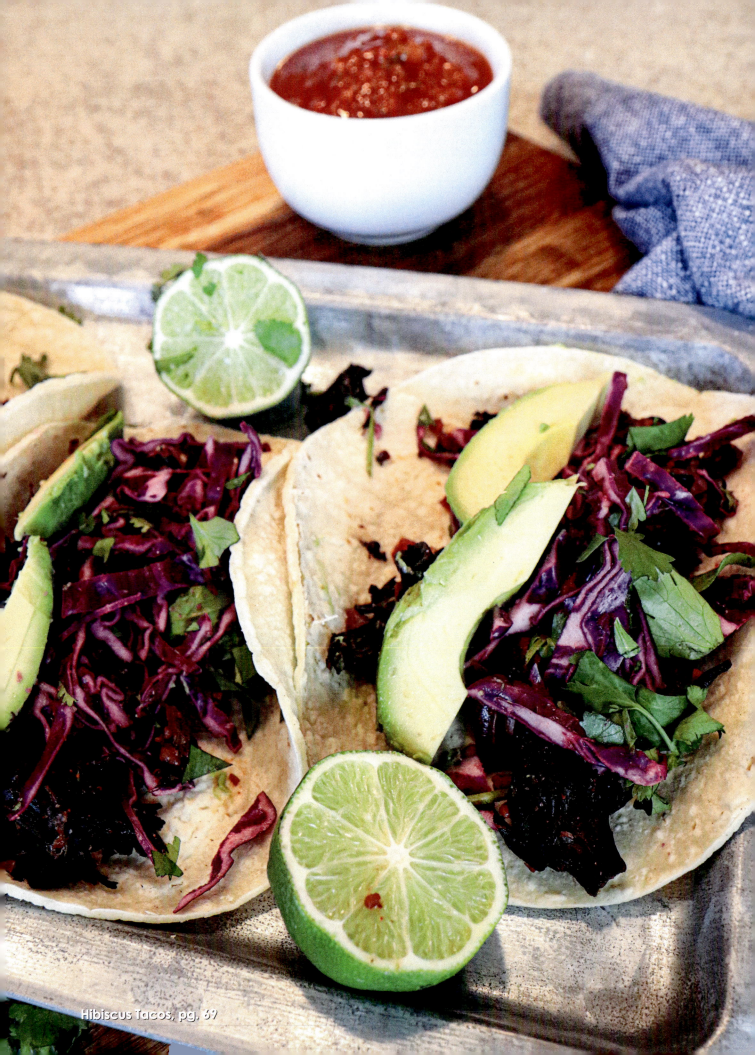

Hibiscus Tacos, pg. 89

THE CALORIE DENSITY CHART

Calorie density defines how CONCENTRATED a food is. It is usually measured as calories per pound. But you could also think of it as calories per mouthful or even calories per meal. The relative difference between the various foods is more important than the unit of measure.

The point of understanding calorie density is to help you consume large amounts of food without consuming too many calories. You don't want to feel hungry all the time by consuming too little volume.

To utilize calorie density to your advantage, eliminate all oils, processed foods, and animal products. Instead, eat freely on a diet of leafy greens, veggies, fruits, and whole starches like grains, legumes, and tubers. Be careful you don't overdo it on the healthy fats like nuts/seeds/avocado/soy if weight loss is your goal.

Using this calorie density "hack," you can begin each meal with a salad or soup to fill up on foods that are more calorie dilute before moving on to more calorie dense foods like cooked starches and whole fats.

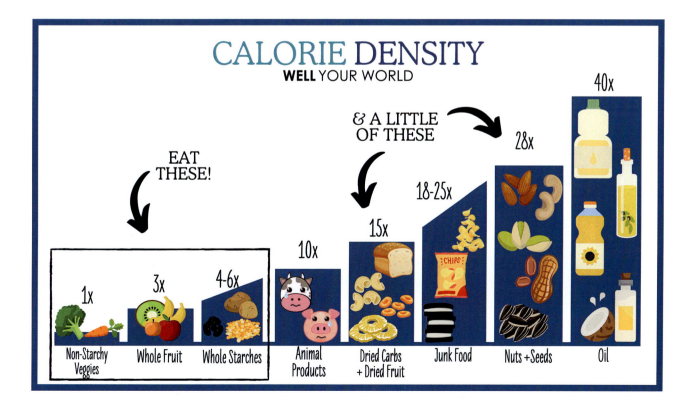

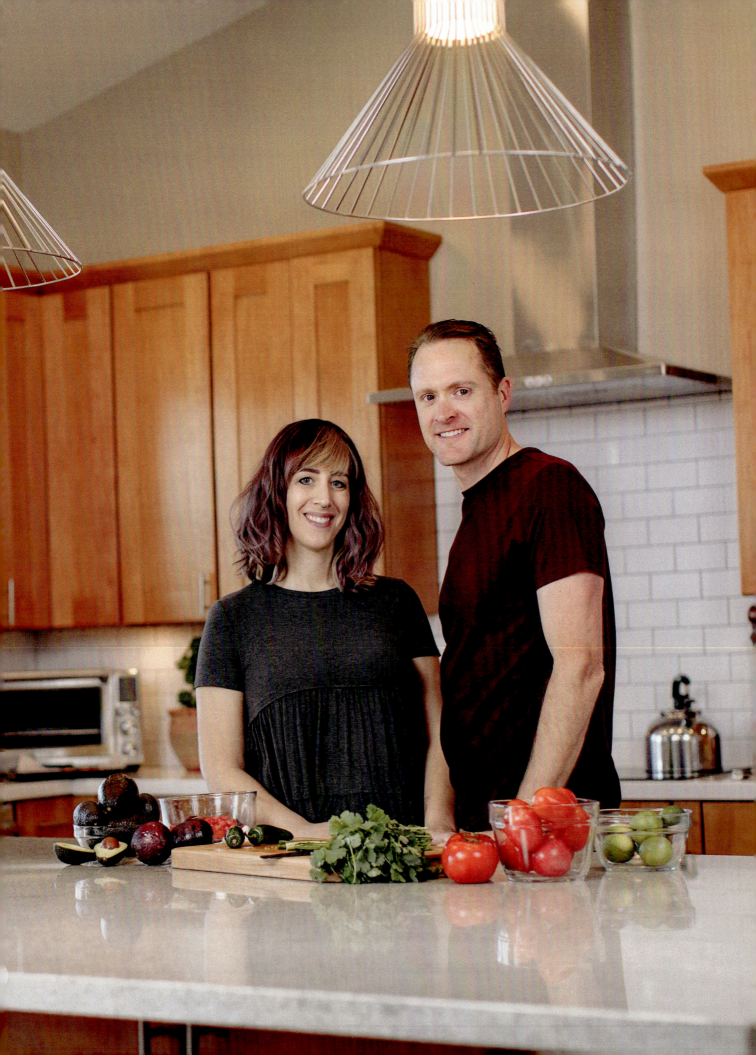

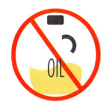 # HOW TO COOK WITHOUT OIL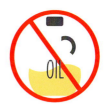

Oil is common for most people on a Standard American Diet (SAD) as a way to flavor, cook, bake, and prepare food. What most people don't understand is that oil is not a health food. In fact, processed oils are actually detrimental to your health.

1. OIL IS CALORIE DENSE

Processed and extracted oil is the most calorie dense food in the world. This includes all oil even avocado, coconut, olive, sesame, etc. Oil is 40x more calorie dense than non-starchy veggies. For example, in one pound of vegetables there are roughly 100 calories, while one pound of oil contains 4,000 calories. Eating oil makes it very hard to control your weight.

2. OIL IS DISGUSTING TO COOK WITH

Oil is simply gross to cook with. It splatters everywhere, stains your clothes, and eventually coats your kitchen surfaces (like the range hood over your stove) in a film that attracts and holds dust. It is difficult and inconvenient to clean up this mess whether it's on your surfaces, dishes, or kitchen walls. Most of us don't realize all this until we cut out the oil!

3. OIL IS HARMFUL TO YOUR HEALTH

Oil isn't just fattening and calorie-dense; it actually harms your health. Many people are under the assumption that type 2 diabetes is caused by excess sugar. While we do agree that refined sugar should also be eliminated from your diet, it's actually excess fat intake that creates insulin resistance in the body, which leads to T2 diabetes. And oil is pure fat.

4. OIL IS HARMFUL TO YOUR HEART

Not only is oil bad for overall health, but it's horrible for heart health. Oil clogs your arteries, which can choke your heart, and eventually kill you. If you have heart disease and eat a plant-based, oil-free diet then there's a good chance you can not only halt its progression but actually reverse it. Most people have less chest pain in only a few days.

5. OIL IS UNNATURAL AND HIGHLY PROCESSED

People like the taste of oil-rich foods because they take advantage of our body's evolutionary mechanism to seek calorie-dense foods, which would help us survive during times when food was in limited supply for long intervals throughout our ancient history. If you want a richer flavor from fat in your foods, focus on the whole, natural fats that we actually did eat throughout our natural history, such as nuts, seeds, and avocados.

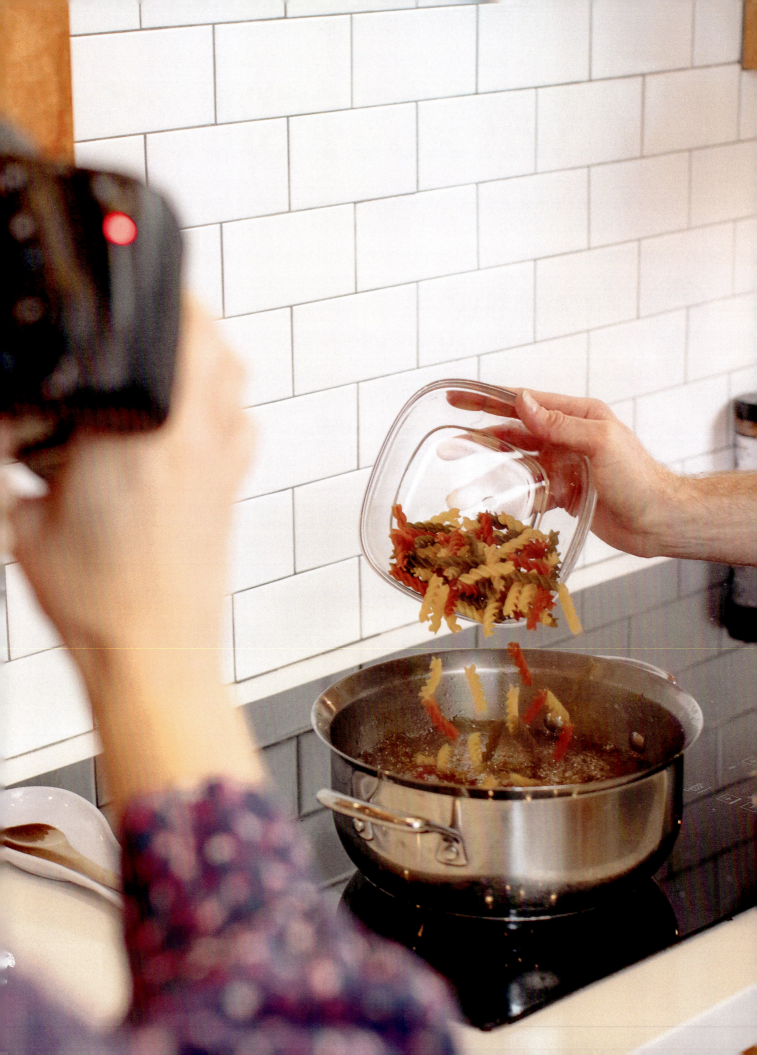

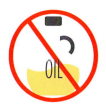 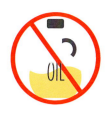

HOW TO COOK WITHOUT OIL

Cooking without oil may seem daunting, but once you learn the basics and get the hang of it, it will become second nature! Here are the ways we cook without using any processed oil at all!

1. SAUTÉING

Throw the ingredients in a pan, add a couple tablespoons of hot water or veggie stock, and stir over medium high heat. Once it dries out add more liquid and repeat the process 2-3 times.

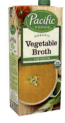 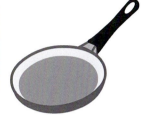

2. ROASTING

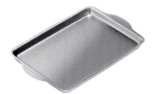 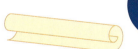

Toss the food with any seasonings and a little liquid to coat. Line a sheet pan with parchment paper or a silicone baking mat, spread around your ingredients, and roast!

3. NON-STICK GRIDDLING

The key to flipping the perfect pancake or making golden hash browns without oil is to use an electric non-stick griddle! Be careful not to use metal utensils.

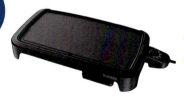

ANY INEXPENSIVE NON-STICK GRIDDLE WILL DO!

4. MAKING SAUCES & DRESSINGS

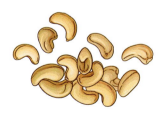 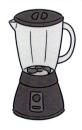

To create tasty sauces and dressings without oil, use whole fats like nuts, seeds, or avocado and blend in a high speed blender. For a lower fat option, white beans work great instead!

5. BAKING & AIR-FRYING

When baking you can replace oil with applesauce, bananas, or even plant milk. To get the crispiest potatoes or fries, refrigerate cooked potatoes then air fry.

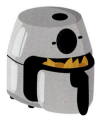 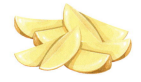

BOOK RECOMMENDATIONS

There are several excellent books that dive deeper into some of the science that supports why a plant-based diet is the number one diet for health and longevity. Here are a few of our favorites, if you are in search of some additional reading.

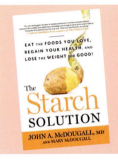

"The Starch Solution" is the book that singlehandedly convinced both of us to try a plant-based diet. It is a very easy read, but also jam-packed with information. It is a definite eye-opener and explains why we should not be vilifying healthy whole carbs.

"The Pleasure Trap" is one of my favorite books because it explains why we are drawn to calorie dense food. Once you understand the process of breaking free of the pleasure trap, you can begin to adapt it to your forever diet, lifestyle, and environment.

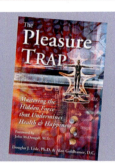

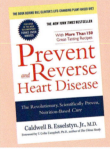

This book is the gold-standard for disease reversal. It is a must-read if you have had any heart-related issues. As always, please consult with your doctor before beginning any medical treatment.

Dr. T. Colin Campbell is famous for railing against the reductionist approach to health in his book "Whole." Rather than chasing after every single little nutrient in our food or trying to hack our health, Dr. Campbell teaches us that real health comes from eating a wide variety of whole, natural plant foods.

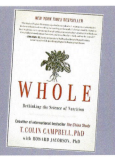

HANDY KITCHEN GADGETS

For those of you who don't know us, we *kinda* have a lot of gadgets. Name a kitchen gadget, we probably carry two of them. While eating healthy and simple doesn't actually require any fancy gadgetry, we thought we'd list out some of our favorites.

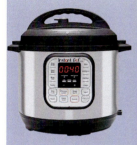

I love the speed and versatility of owning an Instant Pot electric pressure cooker. If you can get one, I highly recommend it.

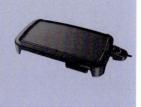

We LOVE this electric griddle. It's cheap (~$40) and super non-stick, perfect for pancakes, veggie burgers, hash browns, and more!

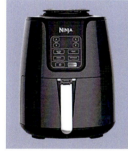

An air fryer is a luxury. If you have one, they are great to use for that perfect crispy crunch.

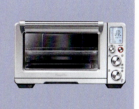

We talk about the Breville Smart Oven Air a lot on the live cooking show. It's a great, compact do-it-all, but it's a bit pricey.

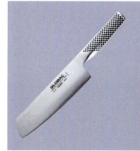

Global Knives are a bit pricey but they are Dillon's go-to. Any decent, sharpened knife is all you need to enjoy slicing and dicing.

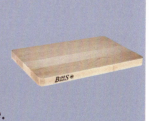

Investing in a really great wood cutting board can make a difference in your kitchen. Take good care of it and it will last a very long time.

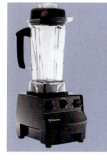

A Vitamix is a high-speed blender that is better than all the others. They have an excellent warranty and are well worth the investment.

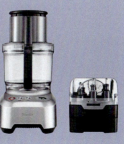

A food processor can really save time in the kitchen, and works a bit differently than a blender. We love our Breville Sous Chef.

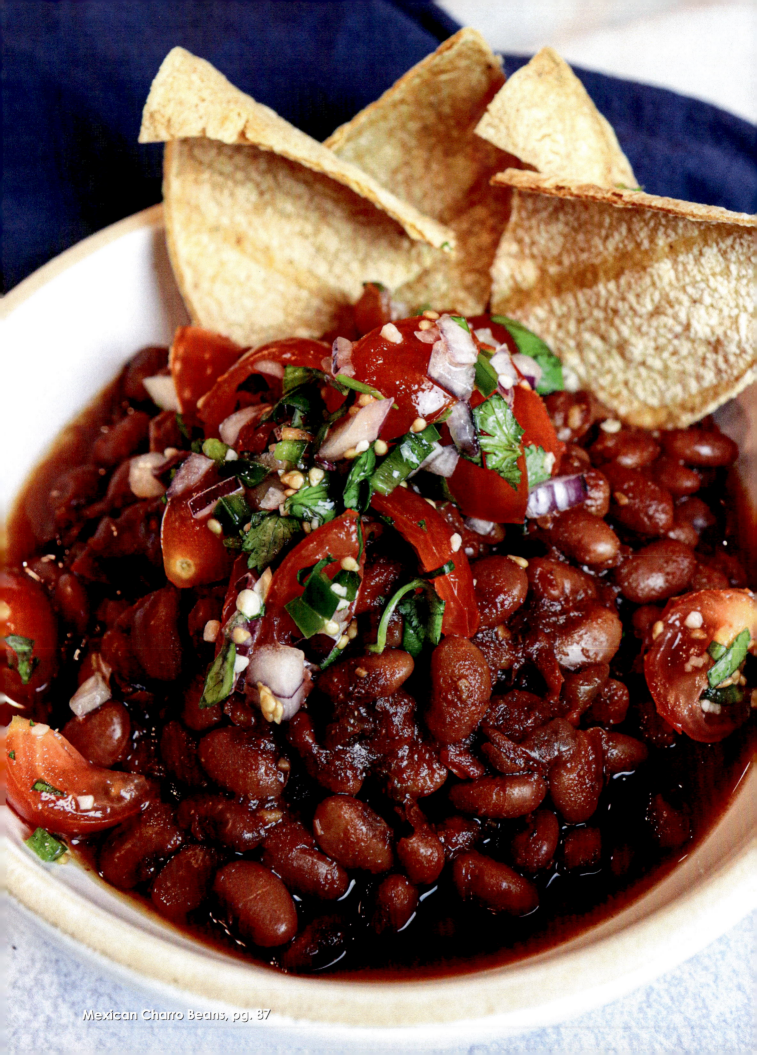
Mexican Charro Beans, pg. 87

RECIPE TIPS & GUIDE

Any recipes requiring plant milk in our book will call for soy milk because it's our absolute favorite. If you are allergic to soy or prefer a different plant milk, feel free to substitute with any milk of your choice.

Dates are a go-to for sweetening dishes naturally without sugar. We use deglet dates in our recipes, because they can be purchased very inexpensively at Costco and other stores. If you are subbing for a different date, like medjool, keep in mind that deglet dates are about half the size of medjool dates.

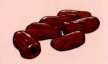

A few of our recipes optionally use soy sauce, miso paste, or olives for a touch of salty flavor. Adding these does add salt to your dish. If you are on a completely salt-free diet, you can omit these from those recipes. All of our recipes are delicious without any added salt.

Feel free to sub your gluten-free flour of choice in any recipe calling for whole-wheat. You can also blend gluten-free rolled oats in your blender to make a homemade oat flour.

We will sometimes use raw cashews and other nuts to add richness to sauces or desserts. If you are trying to avoid whole fats for weight loss, cashews can be replaced with white beans in most savory recipes.

If you want to try out any of our stews or one-pot meals in the pressure cooker, you can! A general rule of thumb is to set your Instant Pot to 1/3 of the standard cook time.

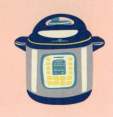

LOOKING FOR OUR VIDEOS?

YOUTUBE.COM/WELLYOURWORLD

There is a YouTube video for every single recipe in this book. The book is named "YouTube Favorites" after all!

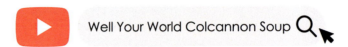

Our recipe videos are easily found by searching YouTube with the recipe name and including "Well Your World" in your search. You can also use the link below to find a playlist with all of the corresponding videos for the recipes in this cookbook.

WELLYOURWORLD.COM/YTFAVESV2

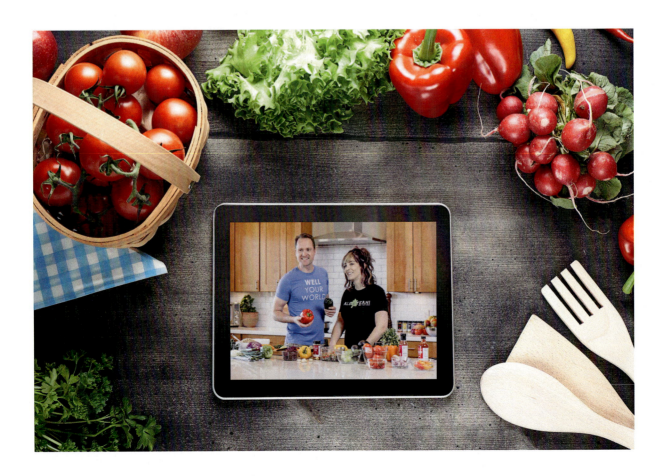

TABLE OF CONTENTS

SNACKS & SIDES
Deviled Potatoes 27

Stuffed Mushrooms 29

Jalapeño Poppers 31

Spinach Artichoke Dip 33

SALADS
Lentil Mango Salad 35

Roasted Asparagus Salad 37

Sheet Pan Veggie Salad 39

SOUPS & STEWS
Colcannon Soup 41

Yellow Split Pea Soup 43

No-Chop Red Lentil Chili 45

Stuffed Pepper Soup 47

Lemon Rice Soup 49

Roasted Tomato Soup 51

MEALS
Butternut Kale Sheet Pan 53

Creamy Broccoli Pesto Pasta 55

Mediterranean Pasta 57

Mediterranean Sheet Pan 59

MEALS
Sheet Pan Tofu Scramble 61

Curried Chickpea Lettuce Cups 63

Buffalo Taquitos 65

Freezer Jambalaya 67

Hibiscus Tacos 69

Instant Pot Baked Ziti 71

Butternut Squash Dahl 73

Baked Beans 75

Loaded Sweet Potatoes 77

Stuffed Acorn Squash 79

Carrot Dogs 81

Tiktok Feta Pasta 83

Quesadillas 85

Mexican Charro Beans 87

3-Ingredient Starchballs 89

Samosa Taquitos 91

Mushroom Kidney Bean Curry 93

Chickpea Omelet 95

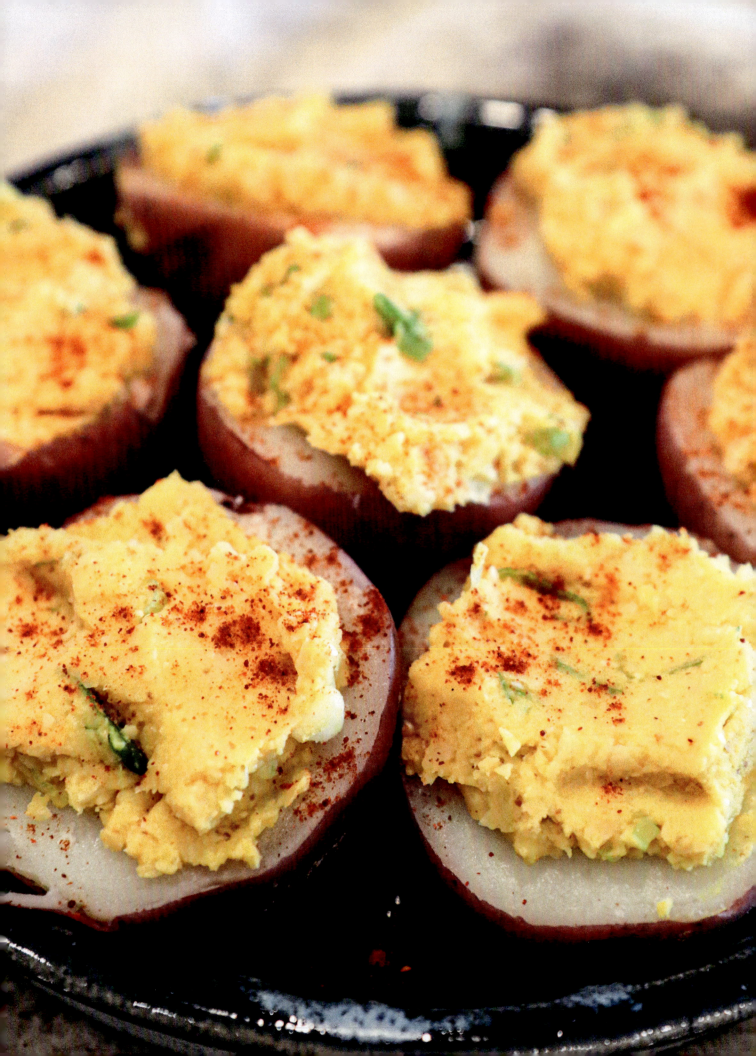

STARTERS

DEVILED POTATOES

You will be the star of any gathering if you take along these deviled potatoes! There's no cholesterol in these so you can enjoy guilt-free!

INGREDIENTS

- 1 15 oz. can chickpeas, drained and rinsed
- 2-4 garlic cloves
- 2 tablespoons lemon juice
- 2 tablespoons mustard
- 2 green onions, sliced
- 1/2 teaspoon ground turmeric
- 1/4 teaspoon black pepper
- 12 small red potatoes, cooked and cooled
- 1 teaspoon paprika, to serve

METHOD

Add the chickpeas, garlic, lemon juice, and mustard to a food processor and process until smooth.

Add the processed mix to a bowl along with the green onions, turmeric, and black pepper and stir to combine.

Cut the potatoes in half. Using a melon baller, scoop out a hole in the middle of the potato. Use the insides for a different dish or pop them into your mouth!

Scoop the chickpea mixture into the middle of the craters you just made in the potatoes. Top with a sprinkle of paprika, refrigerate for a couple hours to cool, and enjoy!

Note: We love making these for potlucks as they can be made in advance and keep well in the fridge.

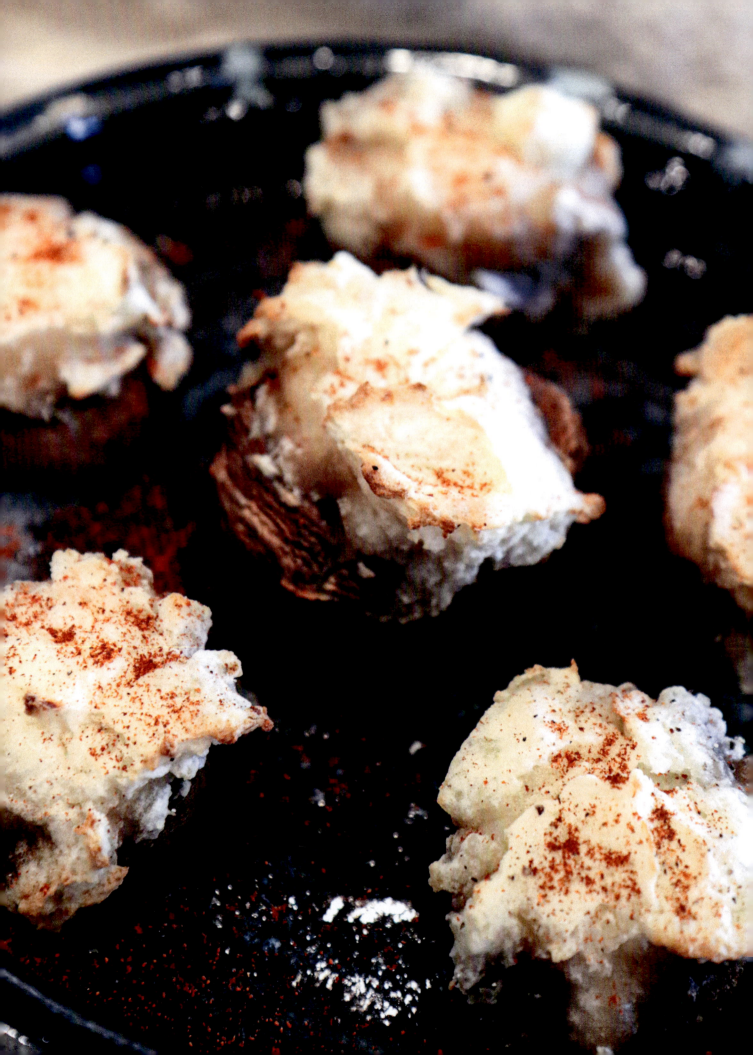

STARTERS

STUFFED MUSHROOMS

These savory stuffed mushrooms are a tasty appetizer to put out at any party. If you love mushrooms, you will love this recipe!

INGREDIENTS

- 6 gold potatoes, cooked (peeling optional!)
- 2 tablespoons garlic powder
- 2 tablespoons onion powder
- 1 teaspoon paprika
- 1/4 cup soy milk
- 8 baby bella mushrooms

METHOD

Preheat the oven to 400°F.

Mash the potatoes with the garlic powder, onion powder, paprika, and soy milk.

Use a melon baller to scoop out the stem of the mushrooms and create a crater in the caps. Using a teaspoon, stuff each mushroom with the mashed potatoes.

Bake for about 20 minutes. Remove from the oven. Serve and enjoy!

Note: Experiment with different fillings for these mushrooms! Sometimes we add sliced green onions or even steamed shredded cabbage to the potato mix.

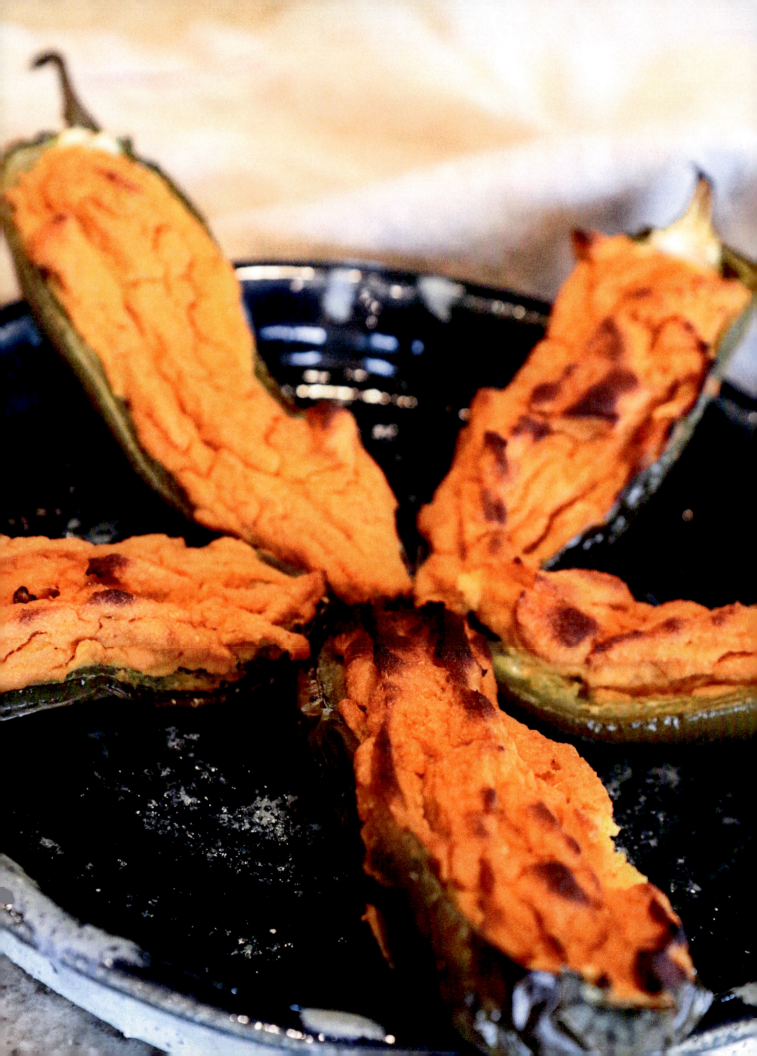

STARTERS

JALAPEÑO POPPERS

What's better than a jalapeño popper? A popper stuffed with healthy ingredients like sweet potato that will leave you feeling amazing, that's what!

INGREDIENTS

- 1 large sweet potato
- 1/4 cup soy milk
- 1/4 cup nutritional yeast
- 2 tablespoons white wine vinegar
- 1/2 teaspoon ground turmeric
- 1/2 teaspoon crushed red pepper
- 1/2 teaspoon garlic powder
- 7 jalapeños, halved

METHOD

Preheat the oven to 400°F.

Peel the sweet potato, cut into chunks, and boil for 10 minutes, until tender. Remove from water.

Add the cooked sweet potato, soy milk, nutritional yeast, white wine vinegar, turmeric, crushed red pepper, and garlic powder to a food processor and blend until smooth.

Remove the seeds from the jalapeños. Spoon a bit of the blended mixture into each jalapeño half and place on a parchment-lined baking sheet.

Bake for 30 minutes. Remove and allow to cool. Enjoy!

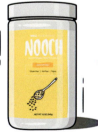

Our Well Your World Nooch is the tastiest non-fortified, nutritional yeast!

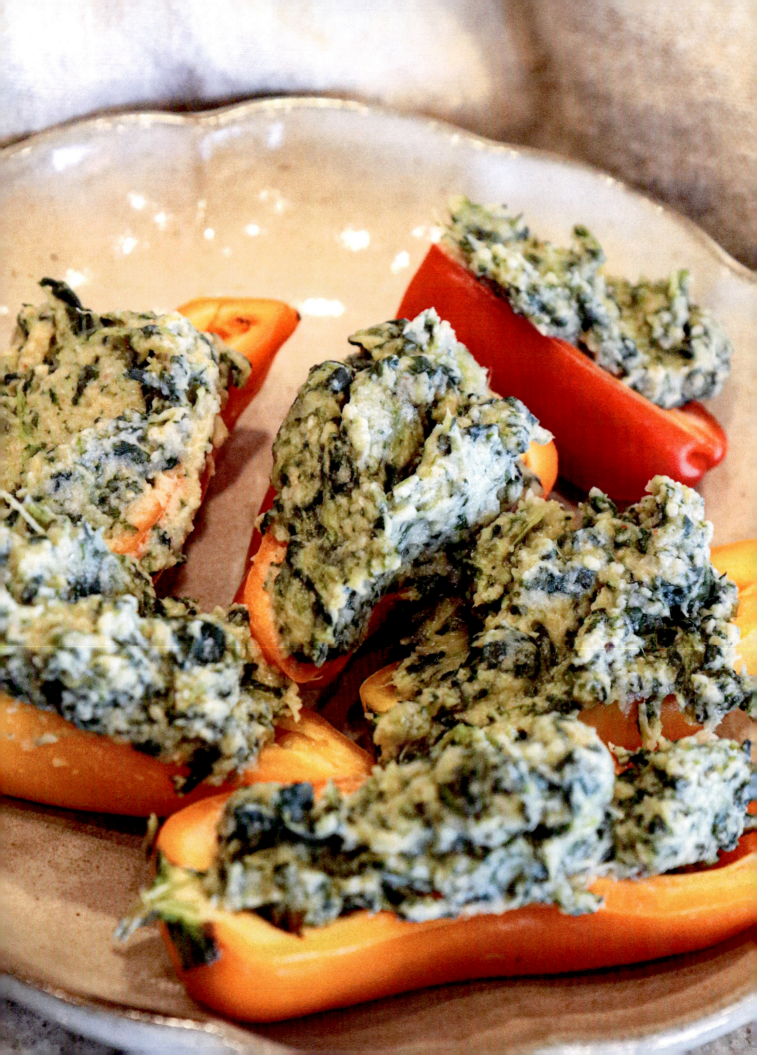

STARTERS

SPINACH ARTICHOKE DIP

This versatile and delicious dip can be used in so many ways. Enjoy with fresh veggies, crackers, or make stuffed sweet peppers like we did in the photo!

INGREDIENTS

- 1   10 oz. bag frozen spinach
- 1   15 oz. can chickpeas, drained and rinsed
- 1   10 oz. bag frozen artichoke hearts, thawed
- 1   lemon, juiced
- 2-4   garlic cloves, minced
- 1/2   cup nutritional yeast
- 1/2   teaspoon chili powder
- 1/2   small red onion, diced
- soy milk, to reach desired consistency

METHOD

Steam the spinach for a few minutes then set aside to cool.

Add the remaining ingredients to a food processor and process until smooth, adding splashes of soy milk as needed.

Once the spinach has cooled, drain and squeeze to remove excess water.

Add the spinach to the food processor and pulse a few times to mix it in. Don't overdo it!

Serve this mixture as is or pop it into the oven with breadcrumbs on top for an extra touch!

Note: Make this a finger food by halving mini sweet peppers and filling them with a couple spoonfuls of this dip like in the photo! This recipe is also amazing with diced roasted red bell peppers sprinkled on top!

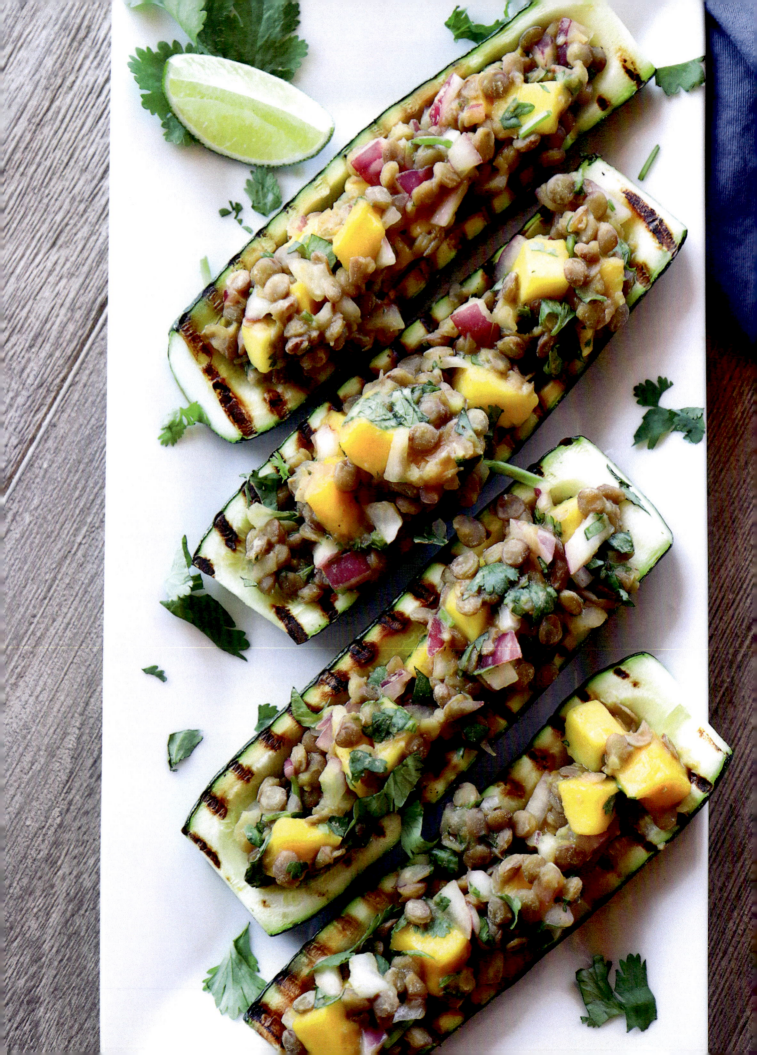

SALADS

LENTIL MANGO SALAD

Our favorite salads are starchy, and this is one of the best salads to make in the summer because it is sweet and refreshing. Serve in grilled zucchini boats for extra fanciness.

INGREDIENTS

Dressing
- 2 cups mango, fresh or thawed from frozen
- 1 garlic clove
- 1 lime, juiced
- 1 green onion
- 1/4" nub fresh ginger
- 10 deglet dates
- 1/2 teaspoon chili powder
- water, to desired consistency

Salad
- 2 cups cooked lentils
- 1/4 red onion, chopped
- 1/2 cup fresh cilantro, chopped
- 2 mangos, diced
  or
- 2-3 cups frozen mango, thawed
- 1-2 green onions, sliced

METHOD

Add all of the dressing ingredients to a high-speed blender and blend until smooth.

Add all of the salad ingredients to a large mixing bowl, add as much dressing as you like, and toss.

Top with additional fresh cilantro and green onions to serve!

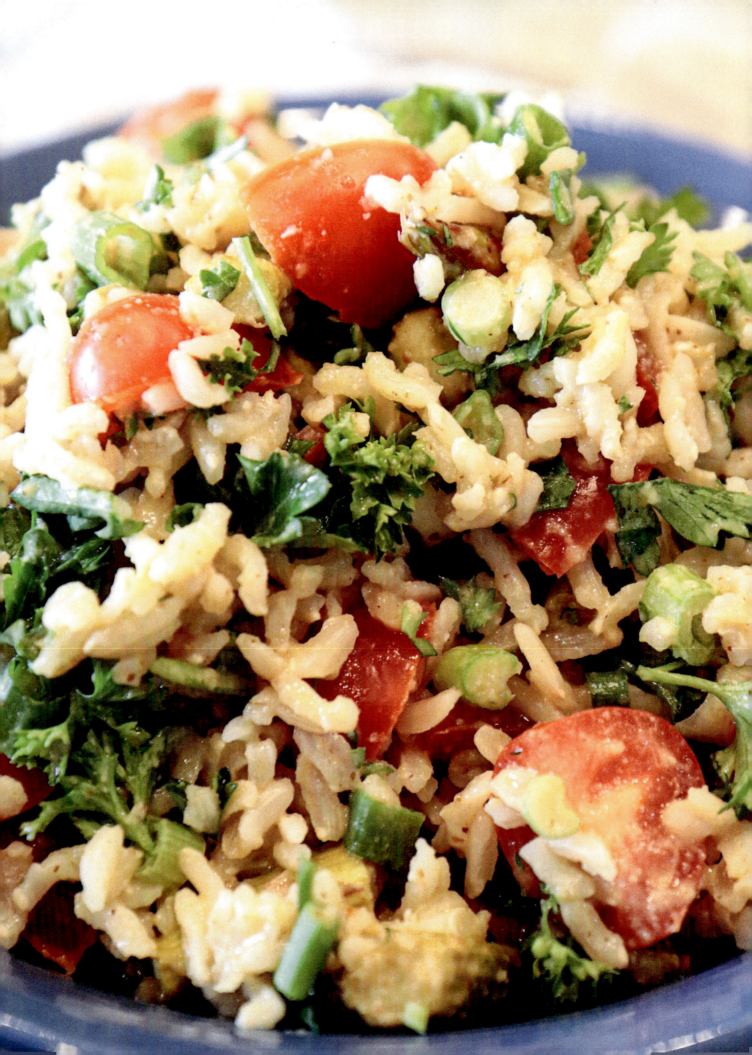

SALADS

ROASTED ASPARAGUS SALAD

This salad reminds us of a warm spring day, as we often take this one with us on picnics! Also, it keeps so well that you don't have to worry about it getting soggy.

INGREDIENTS

Roasted Asparagus
- 1 lb. asparagus, chopped small
- 2 teaspoons garlic powder
- 2 teaspoons onion powder
- 1 lemon, juiced

Dressing
- 1/2 cup white or red wine vinegar
- 4 tablespoons dijon mustard
- 1-2 deglet dates
- water, to reach desired consistency

Salad
- Roasted Asparagus
- 3 cups cooked brown rice
- 1 cup cherry tomatoes, halved
- 5 green onions, sliced
- 1/2 cup fresh parsley, chopped

METHOD

Preheat the oven to 400°F.

Add all of the ingredients for the Roasted Asparagus to a mixing bowl and toss well to coat. Place the asparagus onto a parchment-lined baking sheet and roast in the oven for 15-20 minutes. Remove and set aside to cool.

To prepare the dressing, add all of the ingredients to a high-speed blender and blend until smooth. Set aside.

To a large mixing bowl, add all of the salad ingredients along with the dressing. Toss well.

You can serve immediately or chill in the fridge. This salad keeps very well!

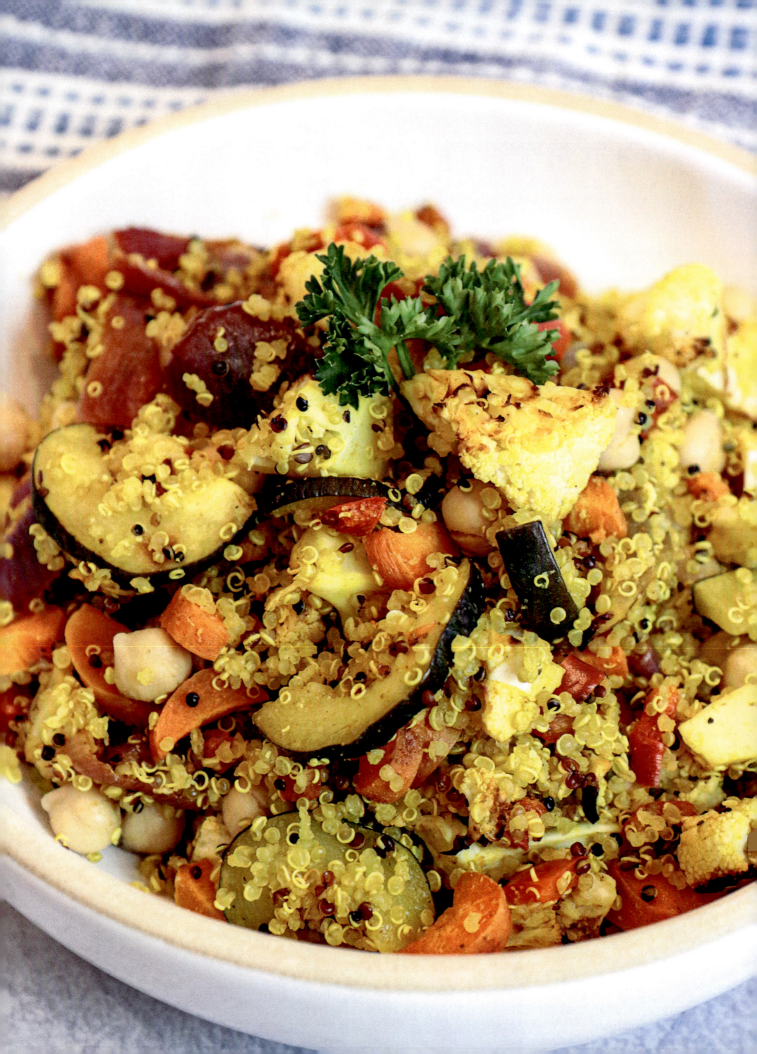

SUPPERS

SHEET PAN VEGGIE SALAD

We love this salad because you can eat it hot right out the oven or cold for lunch the next day. It's delicious either way!

INGREDIENTS

Quinoa
- 1 cup dry quinoa
- 1 teaspoon ground turmeric

Salad
- 1 red bell pepper, chopped
- 3 carrots, chopped
- 1/2 head cauliflower, chopped
- 1 zucchini, chopped
- 1 red onion, chopped
- 1 15 oz. can chickpeas, drained and rinsed

- 1 teaspoon garlic powder
- 1 teaspoon ground cumin
- 1/2 teaspoon ground turmeric
- black pepper, to taste
- 1 lemon, juiced
  OR
- 1 tablespoon WYW Galaxy Dust plus the lemon juice

Dressing
- 1/4 cup tahini
- 1 lemon, juiced
- 1 teaspoon garlic powder
- 1 teaspoon date powder
- 1 teaspoon dijon mustard
- 1/4 teaspoon black pepper
- water, as needed

METHOD

Preheat the oven to 425°F.

Boil the quinoa like pasta with plenty of water in the pot, adding a teaspoon of turmeric to the water to give it some extra color and flavor. Simmer the quinoa for 12 minutes and strain. Then, spread it out on parchment paper to cool so that it doesn't get mushy.

To prepare the salad, add all the ingredients to a large mixing bowl. Mix well to evenly coat everything, then place on two parchment-lined baking sheets. Bake for 30 minutes then set aside.

To prepare the dressing, whisk all of the ingredients together in a small bowl and set aside.

In a large mixing bowl, combine the quinoa, roasted veggies, and dressing. Toss well to combine and serve!

Try our delicious Galaxy Dust Seasoning Blend in this dish!

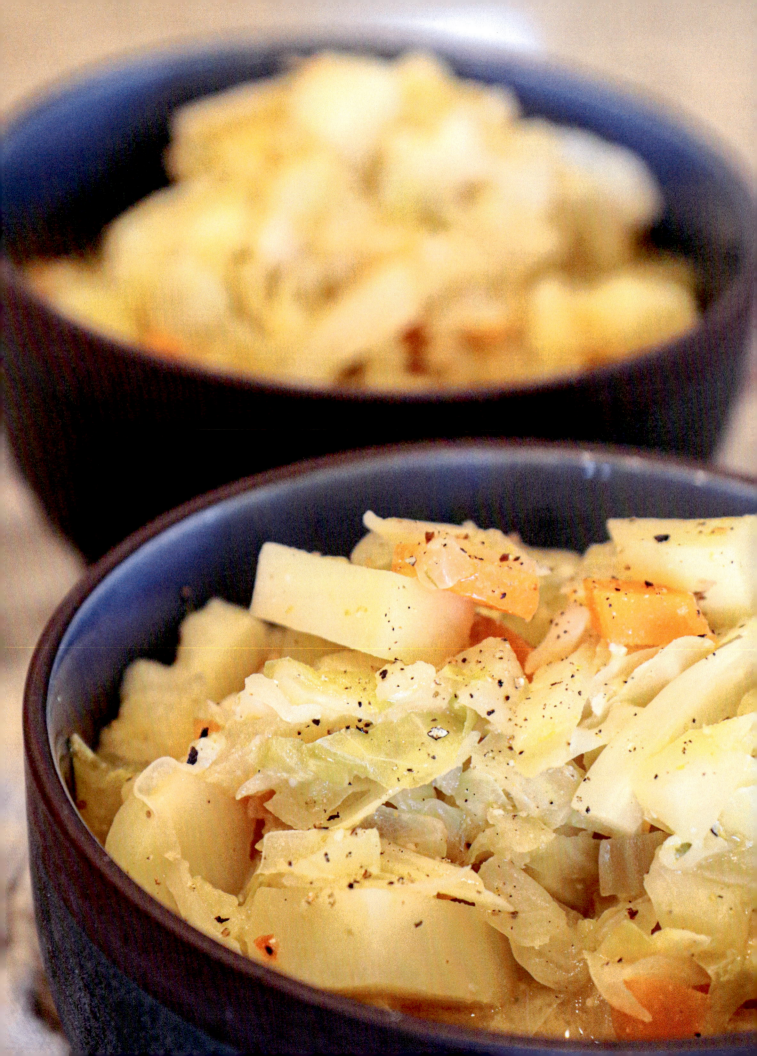

SOUPS

COLCANNON SOUP

This recipe has become FAMOUS in our Facebook group, and for good reason! This soup is full of flavor, veggies, starches, and it's creamy too. Make this soup and you will have enough to last a few meals!

INGREDIENTS

- 4 ribs celery, diced
- 1 onion, diced
- 3 carrots, diced
- 1/2 fennel bulb, diced (optional)
- 5 garlic cloves, minced
- black pepper, to taste
- 1 teaspoon ground fennel seed
- 2 bay leaves
- 2 teaspoons WYW Stardust or salt substitute
- 2 tablespoons nutritional yeast
- 4-5 cups veggie broth
- 3 lbs. red potatoes, peeled and chopped
- 1 medium green cabbage, sliced/shredded

Cream
- 1/2 cup water
- 1/2 cup cashews, soaked OR
- 1/2 cup soy milk

METHOD

In a large soup pot, sauté the celery, onion, carrots, fennel bulb, and garlic over medium-high heat, adding a splash of veggie broth as needed to keep from sticking.

Next, add the black pepper, ground fennel, bay leaves, Stardust, and nutritional yeast to the pot. After a couple minutes add the remaining veggie broth and potatoes to the pot, ensuring the liquid just covers the potatoes. Bring to a simmer and cook for about 5 minutes.

Then slowly add the cabbage to the pot one handful at a time, stirring it in as you go. Add more veggie broth as needed ensuring there is enough liquid to cover the veggies. Bring back to a simmer, cover, set to medium-low, and cook for about 20 minutes. Remove the bay leaves.

To prepare the cashew cream, blend the water and cashews together. Add the cashew cream or soy milk to the pot and mix well.

To serve, grind on more black pepper and enjoy!

Try our delicious Stardust Salt Substitute in this dish!

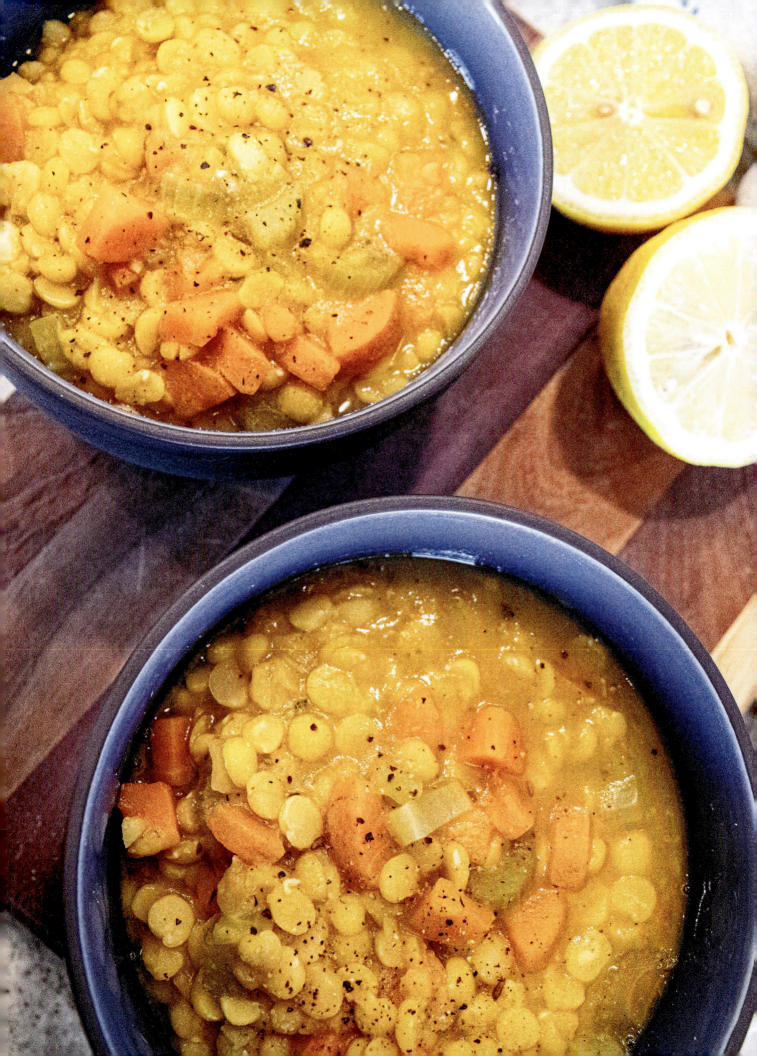

SOUPS

YELLOW SPLIT PEA SOUP

This bright soup is our version Ärtsoppa, a Swedish soup made from split peas. This soup makes the perfect hearty and warming meal all year round!

INGREDIENTS

- 1 onion, diced
- 1 rib celery, diced
- 1 carrot, diced
- 3 garlic cloves, minced
- 2 cups dry yellow split peas, soaked overnight
- 5-6 cups veggie broth
- 2 bay leaves
- 1/2 teaspoon caraway seeds
- 1 teaspoon fresh thyme (or 1/2 teaspoon dried)
- 1/2 teaspoon black pepper
- 1 tablespoon mustard
- 1/2 lemon, juiced

METHOD

Add the onion, celery, carrot, and garlic to a soup pot. Sauté over medium-high heat until tender, adding a bit of water or veggie broth as needed to keep from sticking.

Add the soaked split peas, veggie broth, and bay leaves to the pot and bring to a boil. Reduce the heat and simmer for about 90 minutes or until the split peas are tender.

Next, add the caraway seeds, thyme, black pepper, and mustard. Stir and simmer for another 15 minutes.

Finally, squeeze in the lemon juice, stir, and serve!

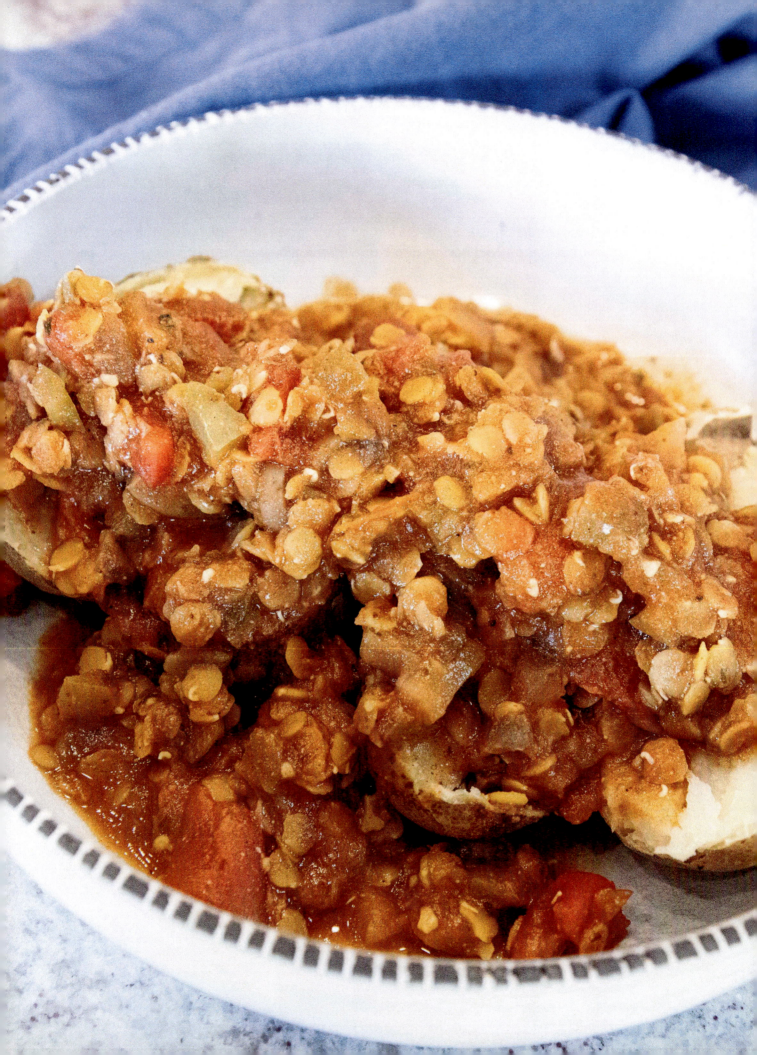

SOUPS

NO-CHOP RED LENTIL CHILI

Nothing is more comforting than a big bowl of chili on a cold day. Luckily, this recipe is so easy to prep and requires no chopping at all, so you can spend more time staying warm and cozy! Enjoy this one on a bed of baked potatoes.

INGREDIENTS

Date Paste
- 1/4 cup date powder
- OR
- 9 deglet dates
- 1 cup water

Chili
- 2 1/4 cups dry red lentils
- 5 1/2 cups water
- 2 15 oz. cans diced tomatoes
- 1 6 oz. can tomato paste
- 1 10 oz. bag frozen onion
- 1 10 oz. bag frozen green bell pepper
- 1 10 oz. bag frozen sliced mushrooms
- 2 tablespoons minced garlic
- 1/4 cup apple cider vinegar
- 1/4 cup nutritional yeast
- 2 tablespoons dried parsley
- 2 tablespoons dried oregano
- 2 tablespoons chili powder
- 1 tablespoon smoked paprika
- 2 teaspoons chipotle powder
- 1 teaspoon ground cumin
- 1/2 teaspoon black pepper
- 1/2 teaspoon crushed red pepper (optional)

METHOD

Mix the date powder and water or blend the dates and water in a high-speed blender until smooth.

Add the date paste to a 6 quart Instant Pot along with all of the Chili ingredients. Stir to mix well.

Close the pot and cook on high pressure for 10-12 minutes, manual release.

For a creamier texture, cook for 12 minutes as this will cause the red lentils to fall apart. For al dente lentils, just do 10 minutes.

This dish also works great in a pot on the stove. Just bring everything to a boil, then reduce the heat and simmer for 20-30 minutes or until it reaches your desired texture. Likewise, this works well in the slow cooker, cooked on low for about 8 hours.

Serve on a bed of greens, rice, or baked potatoes. Enjoy!

Try our versatile Date Powder instead of dates in this dish!

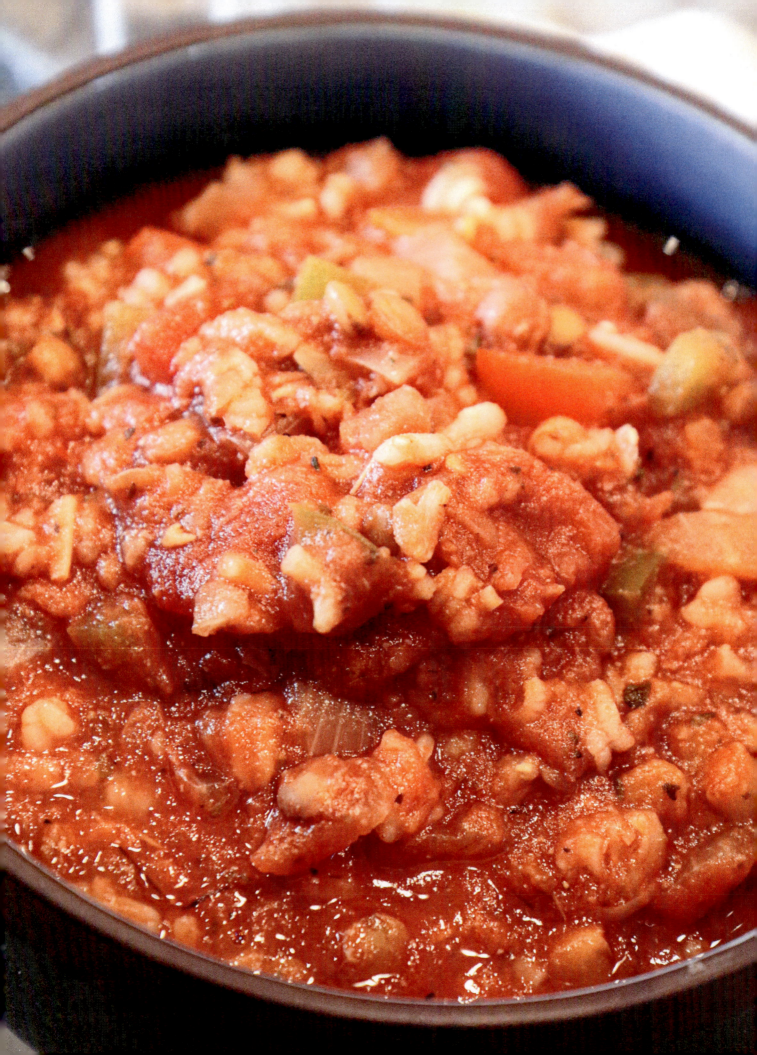

SOUPS

STUFFED PEPPER SOUP

If you love the taste of stuffed peppers, but don't love how much work it is, then this is the recipe for you! This soup has all the classic stuffed pepper flavors but saves you loads of time in the kitchen.

INGREDIENTS

- 2 bell peppers, diced
- 1 yellow onion, diced
- 2 cups veggie broth
- 2 cups lentils, cooked
- 2 cups brown rice, cooked
- 1 15 oz. can diced tomatoes
- 2 15 oz. cans tomato sauce
- 1-2 tablespoons Italian seasoning
- 2 teaspoons garlic powder
- 1 tablespoon nutritional yeast
- crushed red pepper, to taste (optional)

METHOD

Preheat a large dutch oven for a few minutes on the stove. Then add the bell peppers and onion and sauté for a few minutes adding a bit of water or veggie broth as needed to keep from sticking. If you want, you can skip this sauté step and just throw everything in at once for a dump-and-go meal!

Add the veggie broth, lentils, rice, diced tomatoes, tomato sauce, and spices to the pot and stir to combine.

Bring the pot to a boil, reduce the heat, and let simmer for about 15 minutes (or more). Stir the soup every few minutes to ensure it's not burning. Serve and enjoy!!

Note: For a pressure cooker version, just throw everything into the pot and cook on high pressure for 3-5 minutes, manual release.

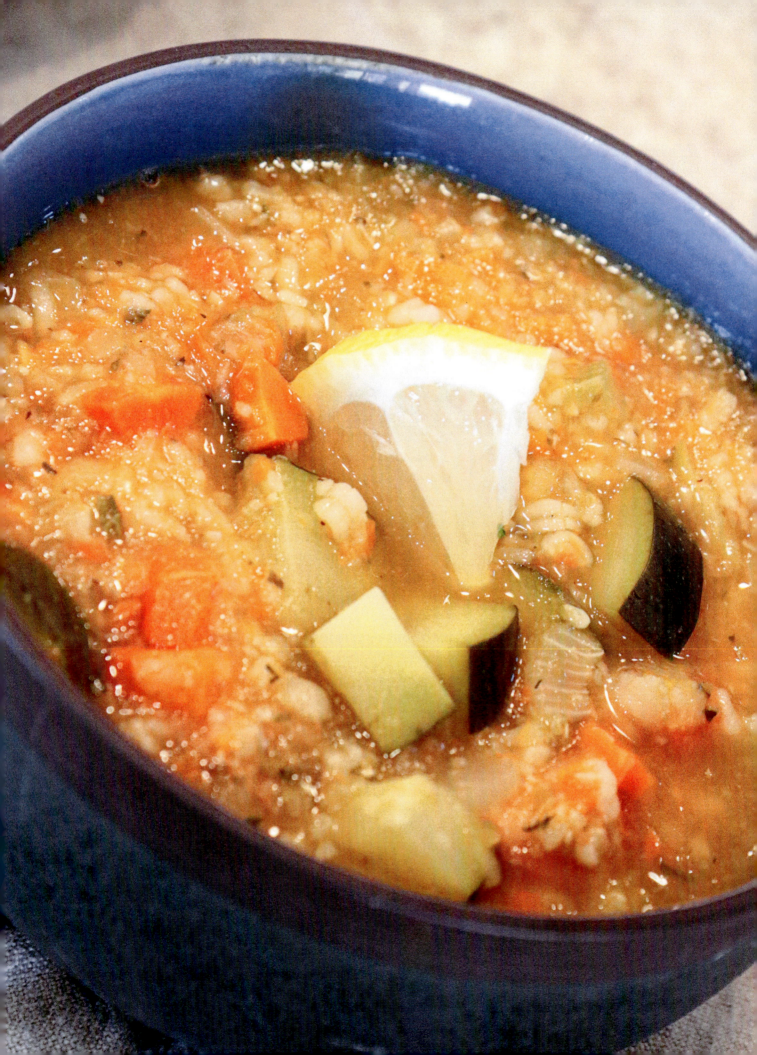

LEMON RICE SOUP

This is THE springtime soup because it is so bright and full of flavor. We use the lemons from the tree in our yard to make this one!

INGREDIENTS

- 1 yellow onion, diced
- 4 carrots, diced
- 4 ribs celery, diced
- 4 garlic cloves, minced
- 1 teaspoon dried oregano
- 4 cups veggie broth
- 3-4 cups water
- 2 zucchinis, diced
- 2 cups short-grain brown rice, cooked
- 2 bay leaves
- 1-2 teaspoons black pepper
- 3 lemons, juiced

METHOD

In a soup pot, sauté the onion, carrots, celery, and garlic until tender, adding a bit of veggie broth or water as needed to keep from sticking.

Stir in the oregano, veggie broth, water, zucchini, rice, bay leaves, and black pepper. Bring to a boil then reduce the heat and simmer for 20 minutes.

Just before serving, remove the bay leaves and add the lemon juice. Use an immersion blender or regular blender to blend the soup to your desired consistency.

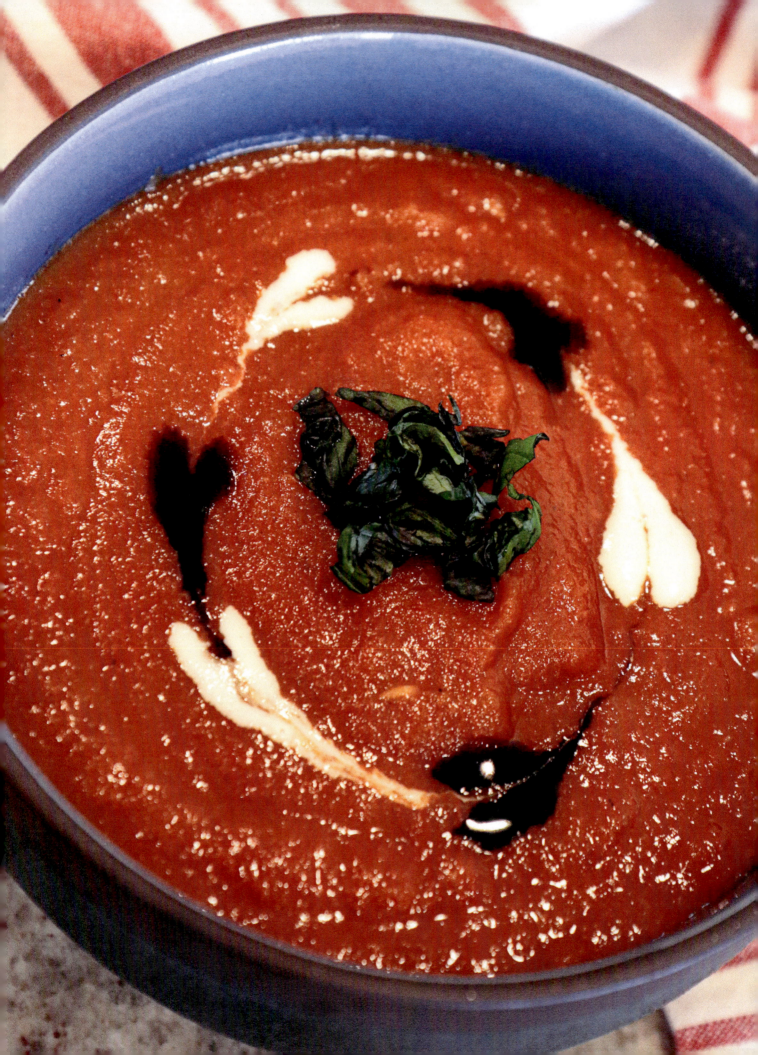

SOUPS

ROASTED TOMATO SOUP

Making a healthy tomato soup is an absolute breeze with this recipe. You can even add Cashew Cream and Balsamic glaze hearts like we did for a fancy presentation!

INGREDIENTS

- ~10 roma tomatoes
- 1 fennel bulb
- 1 head garlic, peeled
- 2 carrots, chopped
- 2 ribs celery, chopped
- 1 yellow onion, chopped
- 1 bunch fresh thyme
- 2 bay leaves
- 3-4 cups veggie broth
- 1 15 oz. can tomato sauce
- 3 tablespoons smoked paprika
- 2 teaspoons date powder
- fresh basil, to serve

METHOD

Preheat the oven to 450°F.

Chop the roma tomatoes in half and spread them evenly in a glass baking dish. Next, chop the fennel bulb and add that to the dish along with the peeled garlic. Roast in the oven for about 35-45 minutes or until the tomatoes show a little bit of char.

While that is roasting, sauté the carrots, celery, and onion in a large soup pot over medium-high heat until tender, adding a bit of veggie broth as needed to keep from sticking.

Now throw it all together! Add the contents of the roast pan to the soup pot along with the remaining ingredients. Bring to a boil, reduce the heat, and simmer for 5-10 minutes. Remove the bay leaves.

In batches, add the soup to the blender and blend until smooth. Then add the blended soup back to the pot. You can cook this for even longer to bring out all the flavors, or just dig in and enjoy!

Garnish with chopped fresh basil and serve.

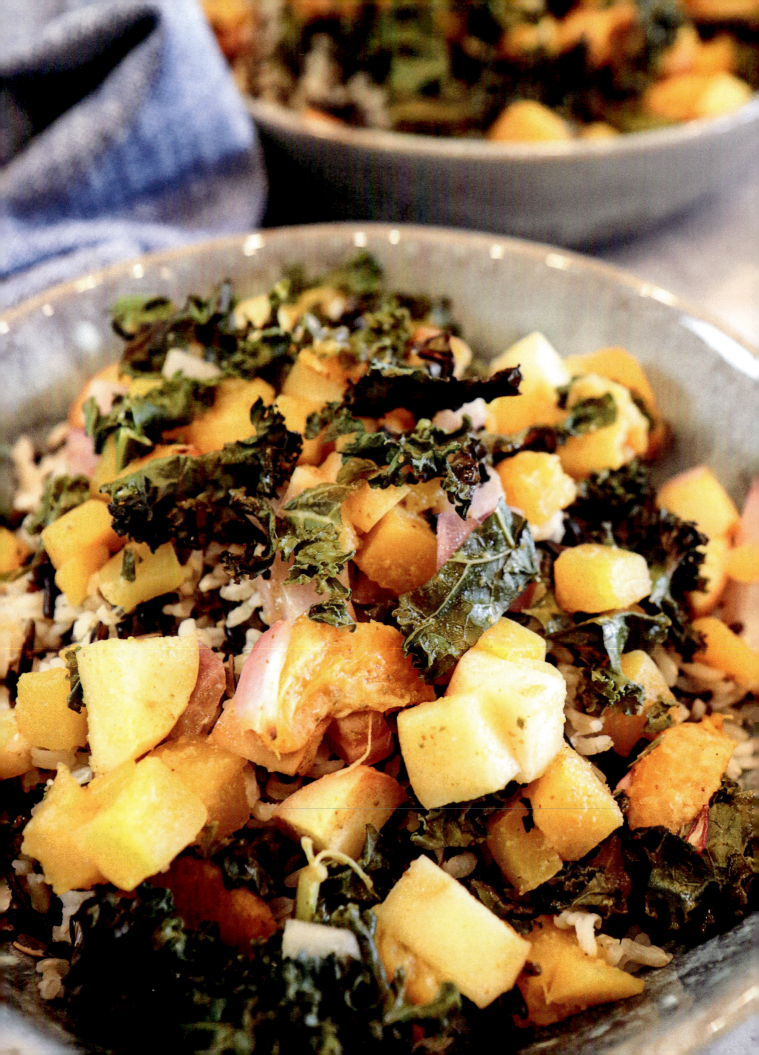

SUPPERS

BUTTERNUT KALE SHEET PAN

This meal is so deliciously simple and easy, yet packs a huge punch of flavor from the zesty fresh ingredients. You'll be making this one again and again!

INGREDIENTS

Vinaigrette Sauce
- 2 clementine oranges, zest + juice
- 2 garlic cloves
- 2 tablespoons apple cider vinegar
- 2 teaspoons dijon mustard
- 4 deglet dates
- 2 teaspoons fresh rosemary

Sheet Pan
- 1 1 lb. bag frozen butternut squash
- 2 handfuls fresh kale, chopped
- 2 small apples, diced
- 2 clementines, split into wedges
- 1/2 red onion, chopped

cooked wild rice blend
OR
leafy greens

METHOD

Preheat the oven to 400°F.

Add all of the sauce ingredients to a high-speed blender and blend until smooth.

Add the butternut squash, kale, apples, clementines, red onion, and as much Vinaigrette Sauce as you like to a large mixing bowl. Toss well and spread on a parchment-lined baking sheet. Bake for about 20 minutes or until tender.

Serve over cooked wild rice or your starch or leafy green of choice and enjoy! Consider making a double batch of the sauce to drizzle on top.

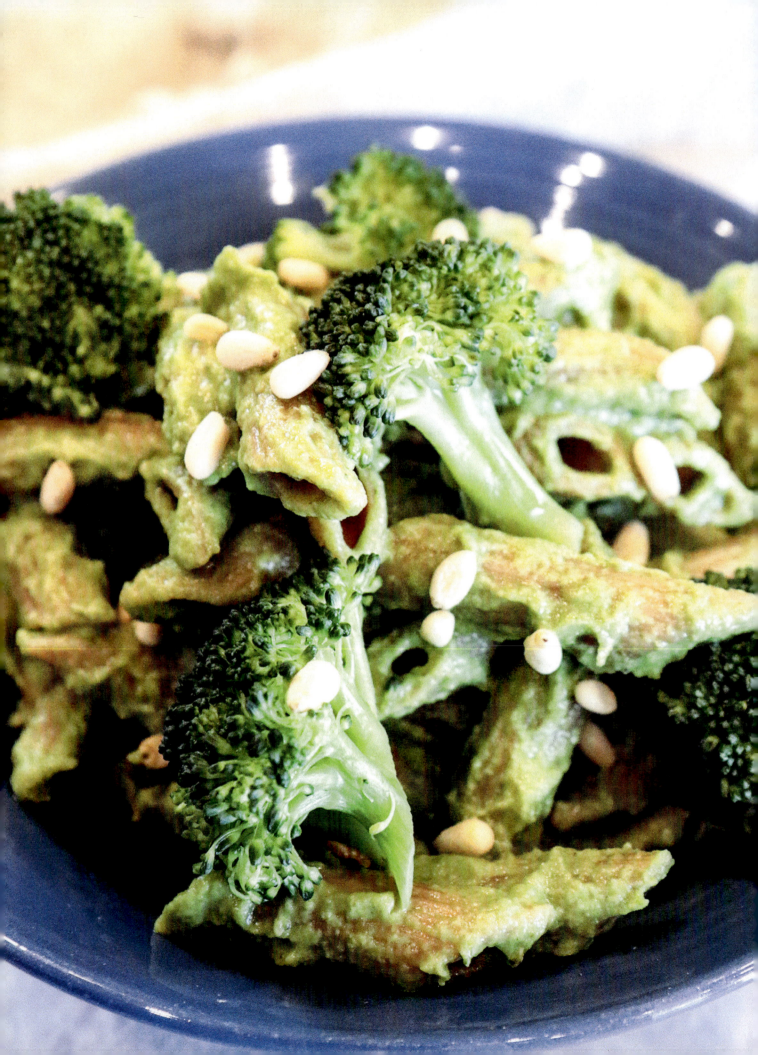

SUPPERS

CREAMY BROCCOLI PESTO PASTA

This recipe is a broccoli lover's dream. Also, unlike traditional pesto there is no oil or nuts, making it a very low fat dish.

INGREDIENTS

- 1 8 oz. box favorite pasta
- 1 head broccoli, chopped and separated into florets and stems
- 1 yellow onion, chopped
- 5 garlic cloves, minced
- black pepper, to taste
- 2 tablespoons nutritional yeast
- 1 cup fresh basil
- 1/2 cup fresh parsley
- 2 large handfuls fresh spinach
- 3/4 cup soy milk
- 1-2 lemons, juiced
- pine nuts, to top (optional)

METHOD

Cook the pasta according to package directions.

While the pasta is cooking, in a separate saucepan, sauté the broccoli stems, onion, and garlic over medium-high heat for 3-5 minutes, adding a little water or veggie broth as needed to keep from sticking.

In a steamer pot, steam the broccoli florets for about 4-5 minutes, or until done to your preference. Set aside.

Add the contents of the sauté pan to your blender along with the black pepper, nutritional yeast, basil, parsley, spinach, soy milk, and lemon juice. Blend until smooth.

Combine the pasta, sauce, and steamed broccoli. Top with pine nuts and serve!

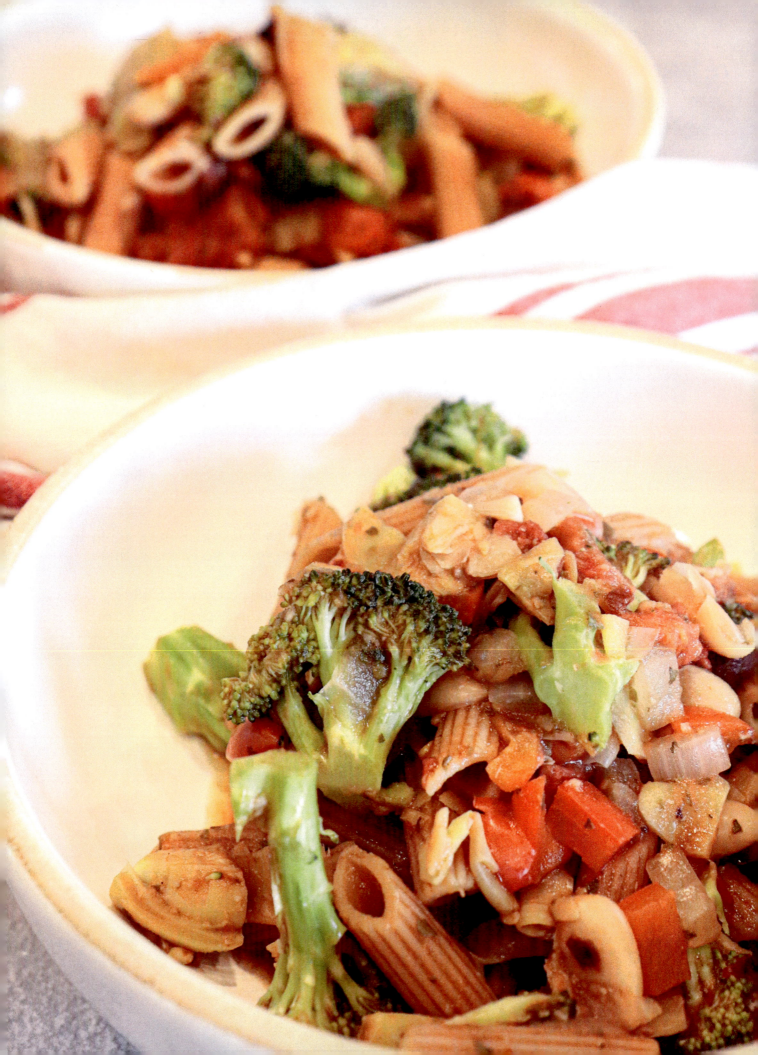

SUPPERS

MEDITERRANEAN PASTA

This extraordinary pasta dish has it all! In one bowl, you can enjoy pasta, veggies, beans, and the perfect combination of Mediterranean flavors.

INGREDIENTS

- 1 8 oz. box favorite pasta
- 1 red bell pepper, diced
- 1 yellow onion, diced
- 3 garlic cloves, minced
- 1 pint cherry tomatoes, halved
- 1 15 oz. can diced tomatoes
- 1 10-12 oz. bag frozen artichoke hearts, thawed and chopped
- 1 15 oz. can white beans, drained and rinsed
- 10 kalamata olives, sliced (optional)
- 1 cup veggie broth
- 2 teaspoons dried basil
- 2 teaspoons dried oregano
- 1 teaspoon crushed red pepper (optional)
- 2 tablespoons balsamic vinegar
- 2-3 cups broccoli florets
- nutritional yeast, to serve

METHOD

Cook the pasta according to package directions.

While the pasta is cooking, in a separate saucepan, add the bell pepper, onion, and garlic and sauté over medium-high heat for about 5 minutes until tender, adding a splash of water or veggie broth as needed to keep from sticking.

Add the rest of the ingredients to the saucepan except for the broccoli and pasta. Stir everything together and bring to a simmer. Allow to cook for a few minutes, then stir in the broccoli and cook for another minute or two until tender.

Stir in the cooked pasta, top with nutritional yeast for added flavor, and enjoy!

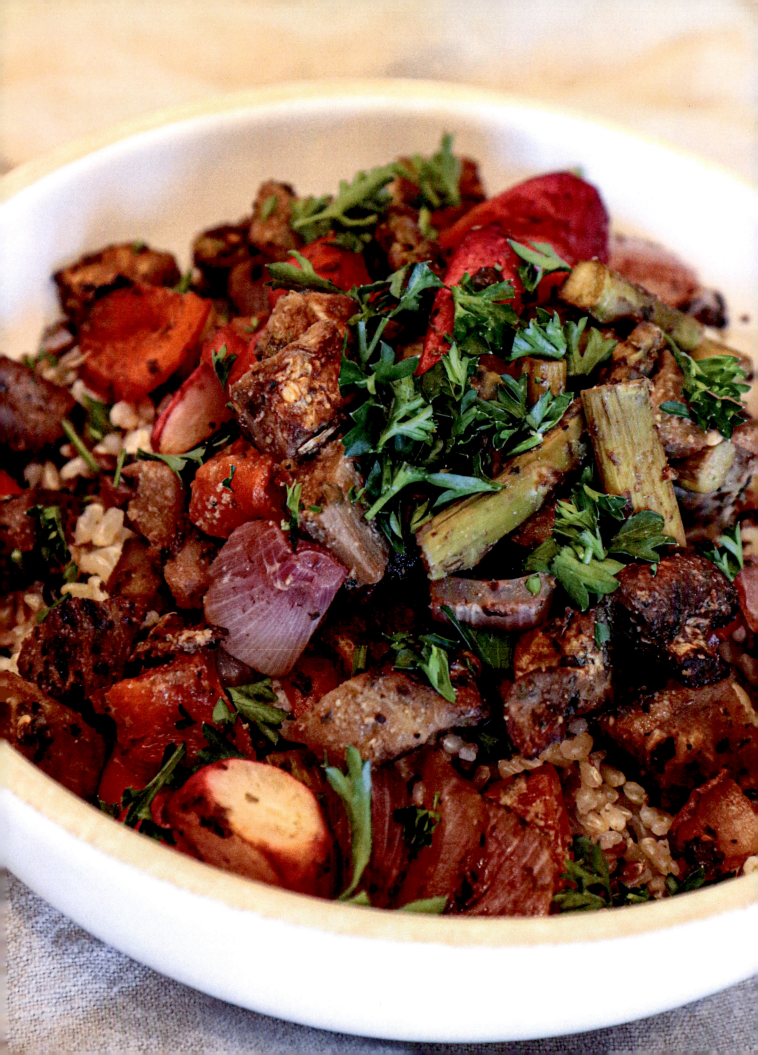

SUPPERS

MEDITERRANEAN SHEET PAN

Don't settle for boring veggies! Try this recipe and make delectable veggies that you can enjoy on their own, for dipping, on a bed of grains, with greens, and more.

INGREDIENTS

- 1 eggplant, peeled and diced
- 1 bunch asparagus, chopped
- 1 large red onion, chopped
- 1 lb. mushrooms, quartered
- 1 bunch radishes, quartered
- 2-3 tablespoons balsamic vinegar
- 2 tablespoons dried parsley or basil
- 2 teaspoons garlic powder
- 2 teaspoons onion powder
- black pepper, to taste
- 2 lemons, juiced
- 1 tablespoon tahini (optional)
- 1 tablespoon tamari (optional)

METHOD

Preheat the oven to 400°F.

In a large mixing bowl add all of the ingredients and mix well, ensuring the vegetables are evenly coated.

Spread the contents of the bowl evenly onto two parchment-lined baking sheets and bake for about 25 minutes.

Remove from the oven. Serve on a bed of your favorite grain or greens and enjoy!

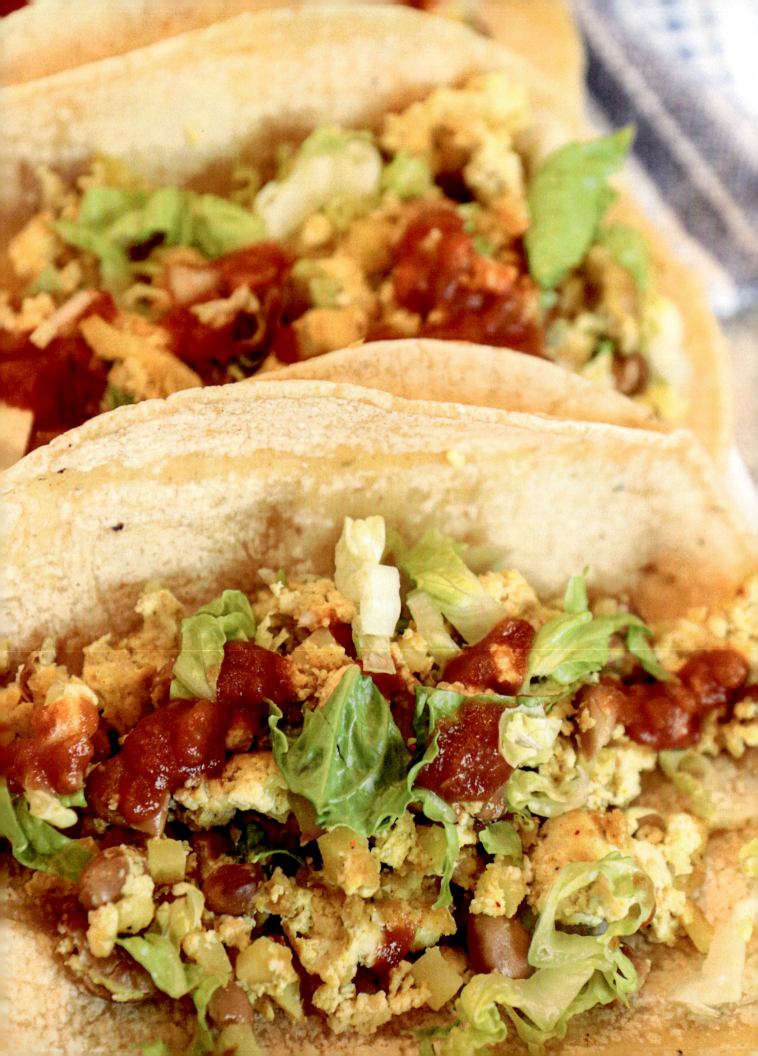

SUPPERS

SHEET PAN TOFU SCRAMBLE

Say goodbye to standing over the stove, because once you make this recipe you will never make tofu scramble any other way. This scramble requires little effort, making it the go-to breakfast recipe for us!

INGREDIENTS

- 1   14-16 oz. block extra-firm tofu, drained
- 1   15 oz. can any beans, drained and rinsed
- 1/2   bell pepper, diced
- 1-2   medium gold potatoes, diced small
- 1/4   cup nutritional yeast
- 2   teaspoons onion powder
- 1   teaspoon garlic powder
- 1/2   teaspoon black salt (optional)
- 1/4   teaspoon turmeric
  black pepper, to taste
- 1/2   teaspoon WYW Chili Lime (optional)

tortillas, lettuce, and salsa, to serve

METHOD

Preheat the oven to 400°F.

Crumble the tofu by squeezing it through your fingers into a large mixing bowl. Then add the remaining ingredients. Stir well to combine and spread evenly across a parchment-lined baking sheet. Sometimes we use two baking sheets for a crispier texture.

Bake in the oven for about 20 minutes. We like to toss on the tortillas layered right on top during the last two minutes, just to heat them up. Remove from the oven.

Top the tortillas with a couple spoonfuls of the scramble, lettuce, and your favorite salsa. Enjoy!

Note: Instead of tacos try this recipe as tofu scramble nachos!

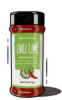

Try our delicious Chili Lime Seasoning in this recipe!

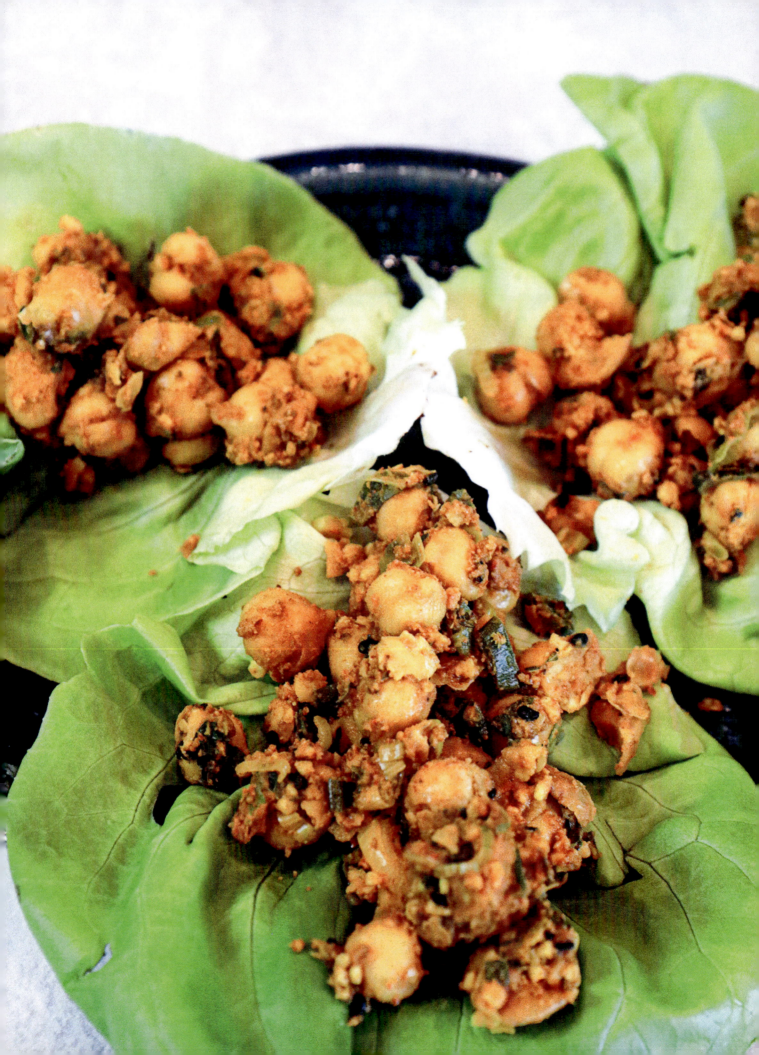

SUPPERS

CURRIED CHICKPEA LETTUCE CUPS

We love any meal that comes together in 10 minutes or less, and this one fits the bill! The crunchy lettuce around the delicious chickpeas makes this meal extraordinary.

INGREDIENTS

- 1 14oz can chickpeas, drained and rinsed
- 1 teaspoon turmeric
- 1 teaspoon ground cumin
- 1 teaspoon ground chili powder
- 1 teaspoon curry powder
- 1 green onion, chopped
- 3 garlic cloves, minced
- 6-8 mint leaves, chopped
- 1 tablespoon sesame seeds

  bib lettuce
  avocado

METHOD

Heat up a skillet on the stove and add a few tablespoons of water along with the chickpeas, turmeric, cumin, chili powder, and curry powder. Stir together to coat the chickpeas well as the water cooks off.

Once the water is mostly gone, add the onion, garlic, mint, and sesame seeds and stir for about 30 seconds to a minute. Turn off the heat and set aside.

To serve, spoon some of the chickpea mixture on to the bib lettuce cup and top with avocado. Enjoy!

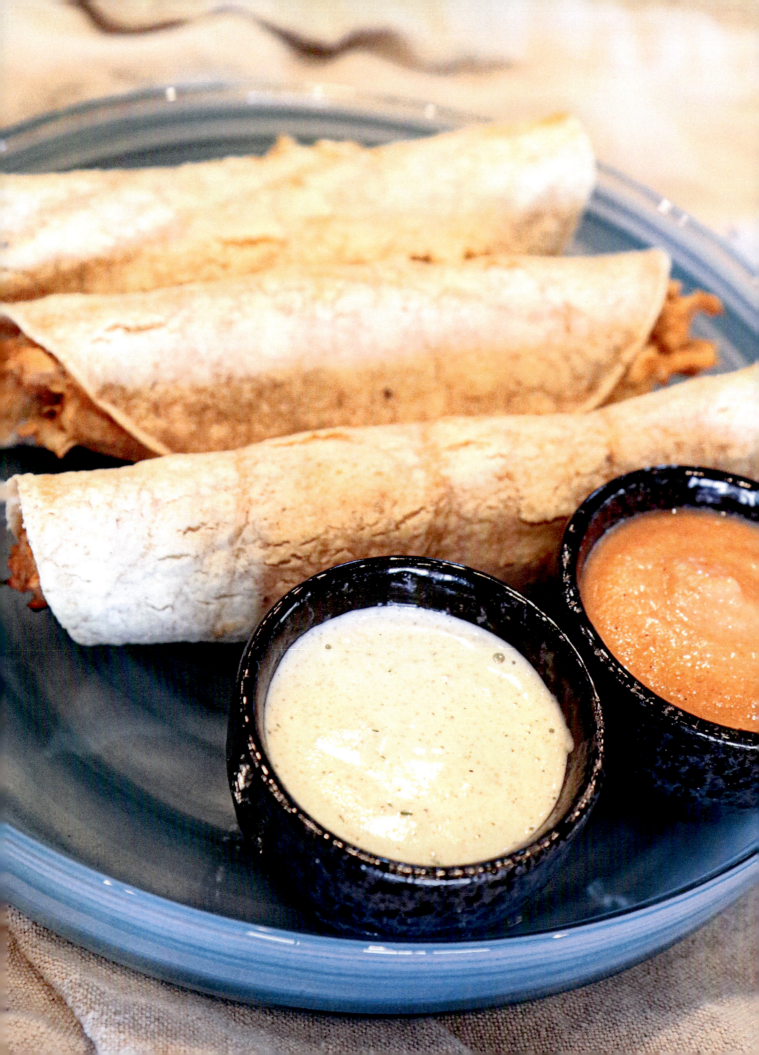

SUPPERS

BUFFALO TAQUITOS

These taquitos make a fun and tasty dish that is sure to be loved by all. Be sure to make a double batch of the sauce, so you have some for dipping! Not a fan of buffalo? Use WYW Cheese Sauce Mix instead for cheesy taquitos!

INGREDIENTS

Buffalo Sauce
- 1 cup tomato sauce
- 3/4 cup distilled white vinegar
- 2 teaspoons minced garlic
- 1 teaspoon cayenne pepper
- 1 teaspoon smoked paprika
- 2 deglet dates
- 1/4 cup cashews (optional)

Taquitos
- 2 15 oz. cans chickpeas, drained and rinsed
- 1/2 cup Buffalo Sauce
- 1 rib celery, diced
- corn tortillas

Ranch Dressing
- 1/2 cup hulled hemp seeds
- 1 lemon, juiced
- 2 garlic cloves
- 1/2 teaspoon ground mustard seed powder
- 1/2 teaspoon white pepper
- 1/3 cup water, as needed
- 1-2 teaspoons fresh dill (or 1/2 tsp dried)

METHOD

To prepare the buffalo sauce, add all the ingredients to a high-speed blender and blend until smooth. Set aside.

Preheat the oven to 350°F.

To prepare the taquito filling, add the chickpeas, buffalo sauce, and celery to a large mixing bowl. Use a potato masher to mash up the mixture into a coarse texture.

Place the tortillas in the preheated oven for about 2 minutes just to warm them up. Then, add about 2 tablespoons of filling to a corn tortilla. Roll it up, then place it seam side down on a parchment-lined baking sheet. Repeat these steps until you run out of filling.

Bake for 15-20 minutes or until crispy.

To prepare the ranch dressing, add all of the ingredients except the dill to a high-speed blender or bullet blender and blend until smooth, adding only as much water as you need to reach your desired consistency. Add the dill and pulse a few times to blend in slightly.

Serve the taquitos with ranch, extra celery, and any remaining buffalo sauce for dipping!

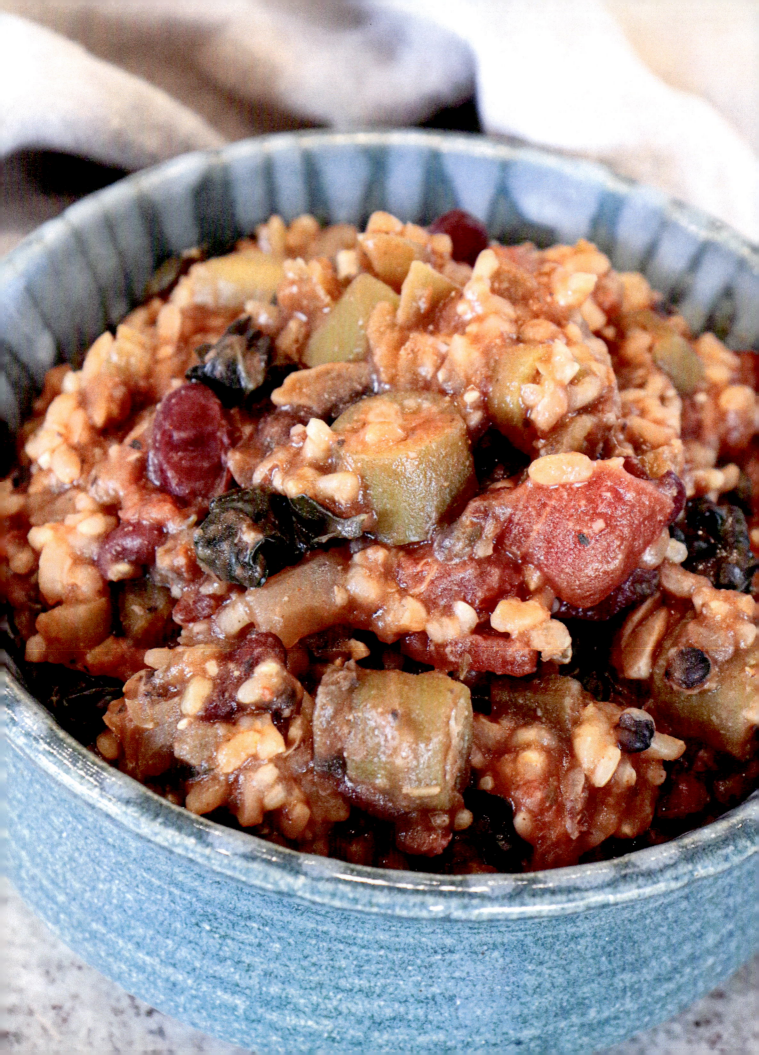

SUPPERS

FREEZER JAMBALAYA

We call this one "Freezer" Jambalaya because most of the ingredients are pre-chopped and frozen. This is a one pot freezer meal that can be thrown together fast!

INGREDIENTS

- 1   10 oz. bag frozen seasoning blend (onion, celery, red pepper, green pepper)
- 1   10 oz. bag frozen chopped onion
- 1   10 oz. bag frozen chopped green bell pepper
- 1   10 oz. bag frozen chopped okra
- 1   10 oz. bag frozen chopped mushrooms
- 2   10 oz. bags frozen brown rice
- 1   tablespoon minced garlic
- 2   15 oz. cans diced tomatoes
- 2   15 oz. cans kidney beans, drained and rinsed
- 3   tablespoons tomato paste
- 3-4 tablespoons WYW Voodoo or Cajun seasoning blend
- 2   cups veggie broth
- 2   bunches fresh kale, destemmed and chopped

METHOD

Dump all of the ingredients except the fresh kale into a large pot or dutch oven and stir to combine. Bring the pot to a boil, then lower to a simmer and cover.

Cook for 10-15 minutes adding the kale in the last minute or two of cooking and stir.

Once the kale has wilted, turn off the heat. Serve and enjoy!

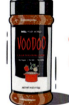

Our VooDoo Cajun Seasoning Blend is perfect in this recipe!

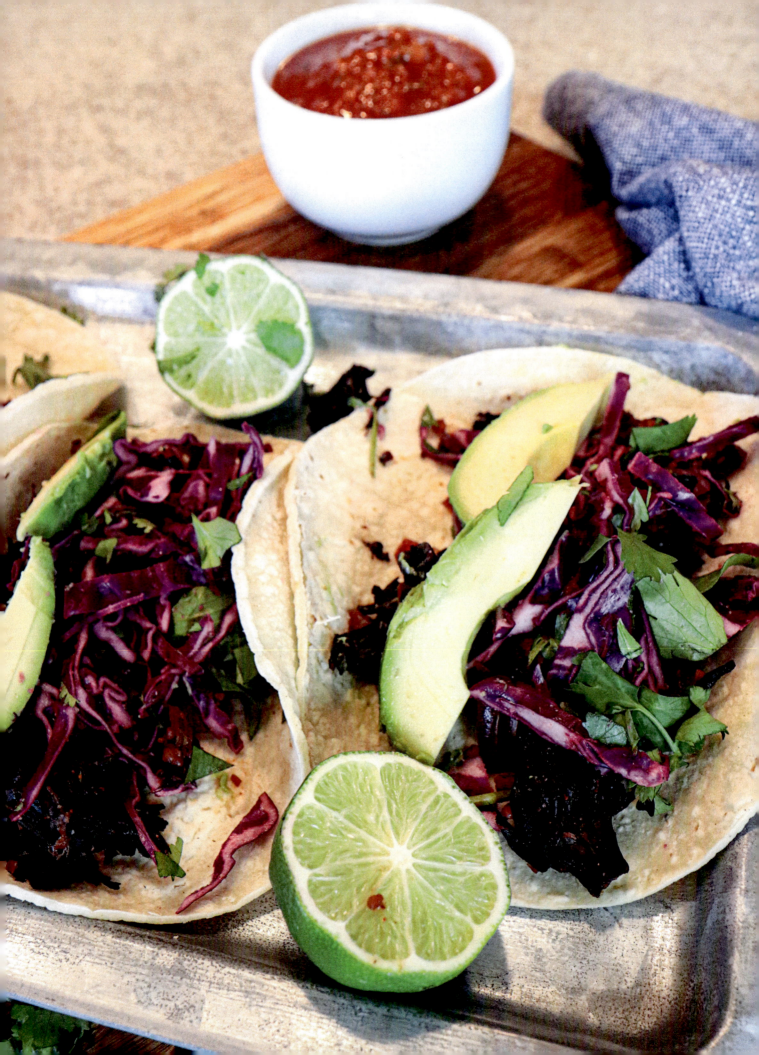

SUPPERS

HIBISCUS TACOS AND TEA

These tacos are as unique as they are delicious! Make these tacos and you will have a refreshing tea to go with. We often find dried hibiscus flowers at our local Latin market or you can find them online.

INGREDIENTS

Hibiscus Tea
- 2 cups dry hibiscus flowers
- 8 cups water
- 1 tablespoon WYW Date Powder (optional)

Hibiscus Tacos
- 2 cups steeped hibiscus flowers
- 1/2 small red onion, diced
- 3-4 garlic cloves, minced
- 1 tablespoon WYW Fiesta or Mexican spice blend

corn tortillas, coleslaw, and avocado, to serve

Coleslaw
- 1/4 head red cabbage, sliced thin
- 2 teaspoons ground cumin or WYW Fiesta Blend
- 1 teaspoon garlic powder
- 1 bunch fresh cilantro, chopped
- 1-2 limes, juiced

METHOD

To prepare the tea, rinse the flowers well in cold water for about 30 seconds to remove any grit. In a small pot add the water and hibiscus flowers and bring to a boil. Stir and reduce the heat to low and simmer for 20 minutes. Turn off the heat, cover the pot, and let steep for 20 minutes to an hour. Strain out the flowers with a fine mesh strainer and store the concentrated tea in a mason jar in the fridge. Keep the flowers for the tacos. When you're ready for a glass of tea, dilute the concentrate with water to your liking, add the date powder to sweeten, and enjoy. WYW Date Powder is best for this because it is ground fine.

To prepare the tacos, rinse the steeped hibiscus flowers again for 30 seconds. Sauté the onion and garlic until tender, adding water as needed to keep from sticking. Add your favorite Mexican spice blend and toss in the hibiscus flowers and continue to sauté until heated through. Turn off the heat and cover.

To prepare the coleslaw add the cabbage, cumin or Fiesta, garlic powder, cilantro, and lime juice to a large mixing bowl and stir well.

Add the hibiscus taco meat to warm corn tortillas along with the coleslaw and avocado. Enjoy with a tall glass of hibiscus tea!

Try our popular Fiesta Blend in this recipe!

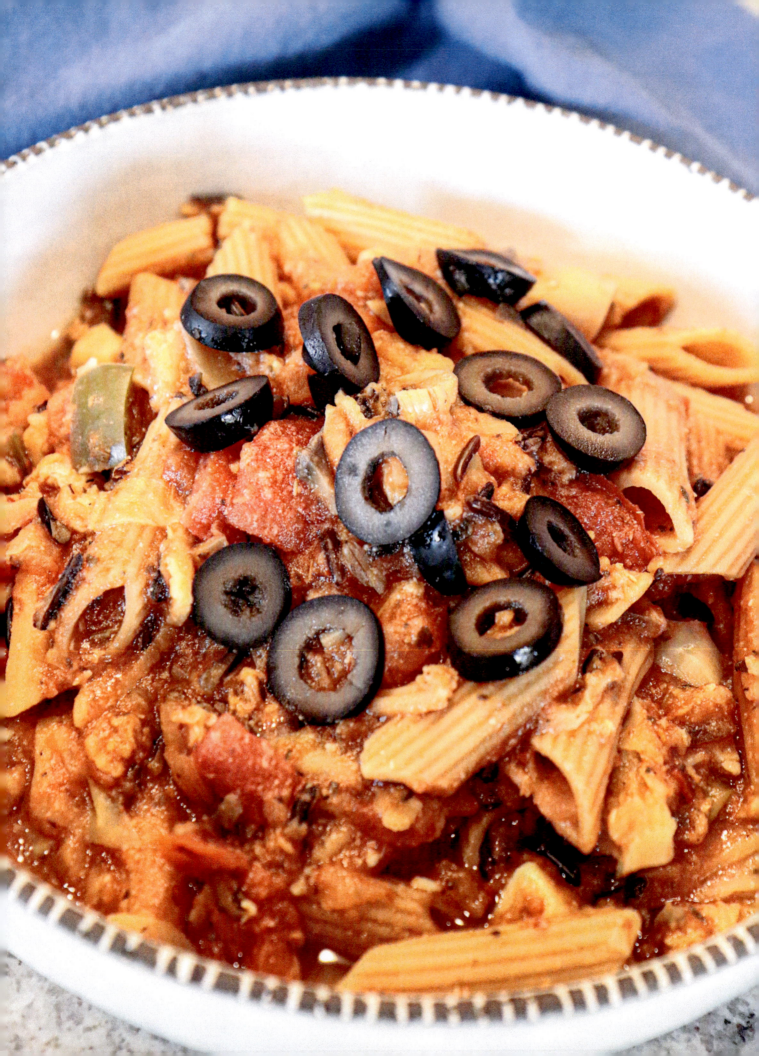

SUPPERS

INSTANT POT BAKED ZITI

With no chopping involved and so much flavor, there's a good reason why it is so popular in the Well Your World Community! Set it and forget it!

INGREDIENTS

1	10 oz. bag frozen chopped yellow onion
1	10. oz bag frozen chopped bell pepper
6-10	mushrooms, diced (fresh or frozen)
2 1/2	cups uncooked favorite pasta
1/2	cup dry red lentils
1/2	cup dry wild rice
1	cup soy curls (optional)
3	tablespoons Italian seasoning
2	teaspoons crushed red pepper (optional)
3	tablespoons nutritional yeast
1	tablespoon garlic powder
2	15 oz. cans diced tomatoes
2	15 oz. cans tomato sauce
1	10 oz. bag frozen artichoke hearts
6	cups water

sliced black olives, to serve

METHOD

Add all of the ingredients to a 6-quart or 8-quart pressure cooker and stir well.

Set the pressure cooker on high pressure for 20 minutes, quick release.

Top with sliced black olives or a sprinkle of nutritional yeast for even more richness and enjoy!

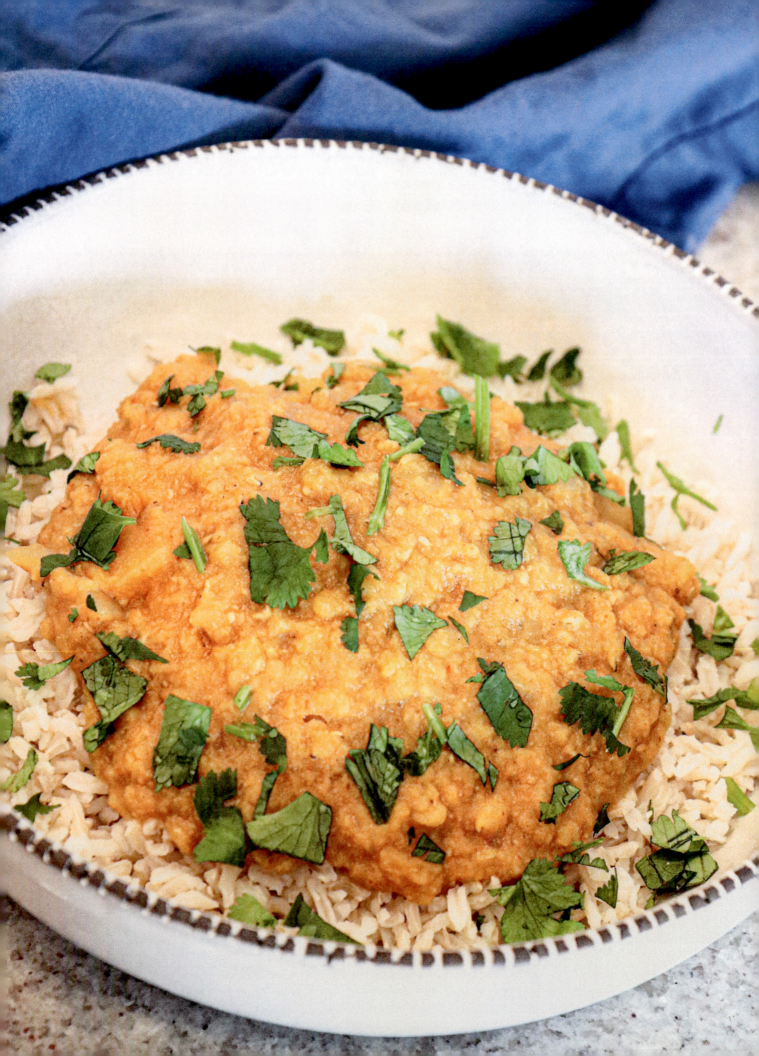

SUPPERS

BUTTERNUT SQUASH DAHL

You can make this Dahl in just 5 minutes in your pressure cooker. This is a go-to recipe on really busy work nights.

INGREDIENTS

- 2 cups dry red lentils
- 1 10 oz. bag frozen chopped yellow onion
- 1 1 lb. bag frozen butternut squash
- 5 cups water
- 1 cup soy milk
- 2 tablespoons tomato paste
- 1-2 tablespoons date powder (optional)
- 2 teaspoons garlic powder
- 2 teaspoons ground ginger
- 1/4 teaspoon chili powder
- 1/2 teaspoon ground turmeric
- 1 tablespoon curry powder
- 2 teaspoons ground coriander
- 1/2 teaspoon ground cumin

METHOD

Add all of the ingredients to a pressure cooker and stir well. Set for 5 minutes on high pressure. Allow to natural release for at least 5 minutes then manual release the remaining pressure. Remove the lid and stir well to smooth out the butternut squash.

Enjoy over a bed of rice or your favorite grain!

Try our versatile Date Powder in this dish!

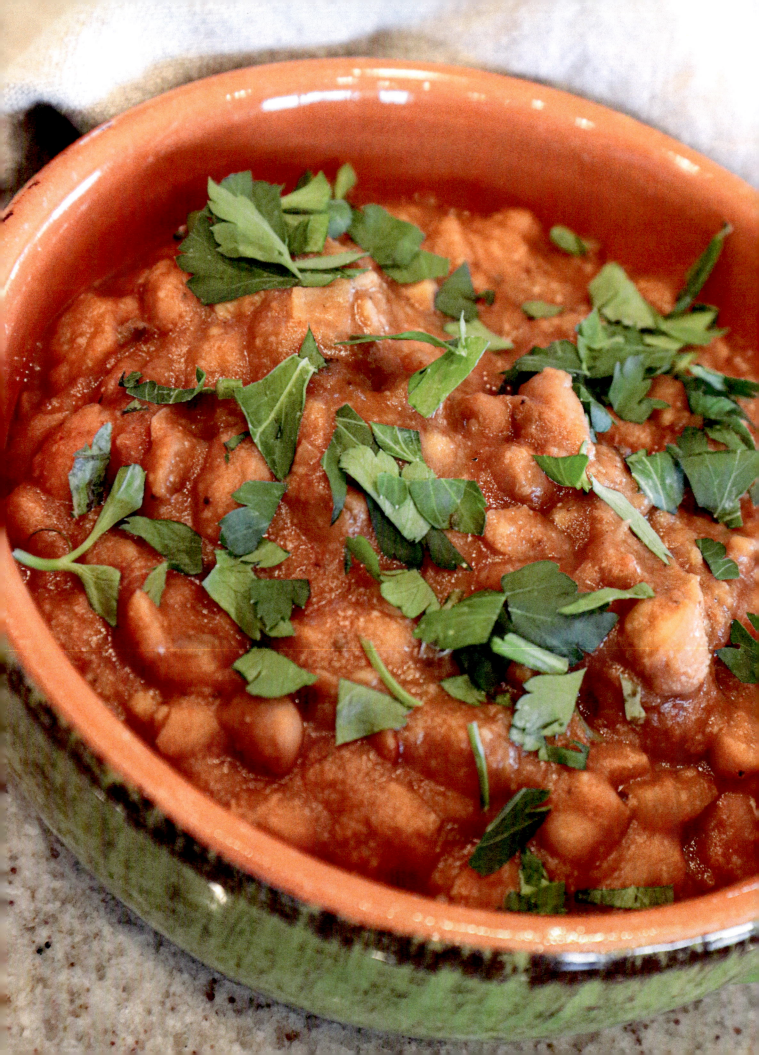

SUPPERS

BAKED BEANS

Enjoy the taste of baked beans again, now with healthy ingredients! What makes this recipe so amazing is that it is sweetened with pineapple instead of processed sugar. This makes a big batch, so it's perfect for parties!

INGREDIENTS

- 1 yellow onion, diced small
- 5 garlic cloves, minced
- 1 1/2 teaspoons ground cumin
- 1 1/2 teaspoons smoked paprika
- 1/2-1 teaspoon crushed red pepper (optional)
- 1 teaspoon mustard powder
- 1 teaspoon chipotle powder
- 1/4 teaspoon white pepper
- 1 tablespoon WYW Voodoo or Cajun seasoning blend
- 1 teaspoon liquid smoke (optional)
- 3 tablespoons apple cider vinegar
- 1 6 oz. can tomato paste
- 4 15 oz. cans pinto beans, with liquid
- 1 1/2 cups pineapple, minced (fresh or frozen)

    fresh chopped cilantro, to serve

METHOD

Add the onion to a large stock pot or dutch oven and sauté over medium-high heat for about 5 minutes or until tender, adding some water or veggie broth as needed to keep from sticking. You'll want to sauté these onions on the dry side to "brown" them.

Once the onions have browned, add the remaining ingredients to the pot, stir, and bring to a boil.

Reduce the heat to low, cover, and let cook for about 30 minutes (or more). This will allow the flavors and textures to come together into the perfect baked beans.

Garnish with cilantro, serve, and enjoy!

Note: Don't have pineapple? Try using chopped mango, dates, or WYW Date Powder instead!

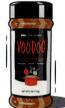

Our VooDoo Cajun Seasoning Blend is perfect in this recipe!

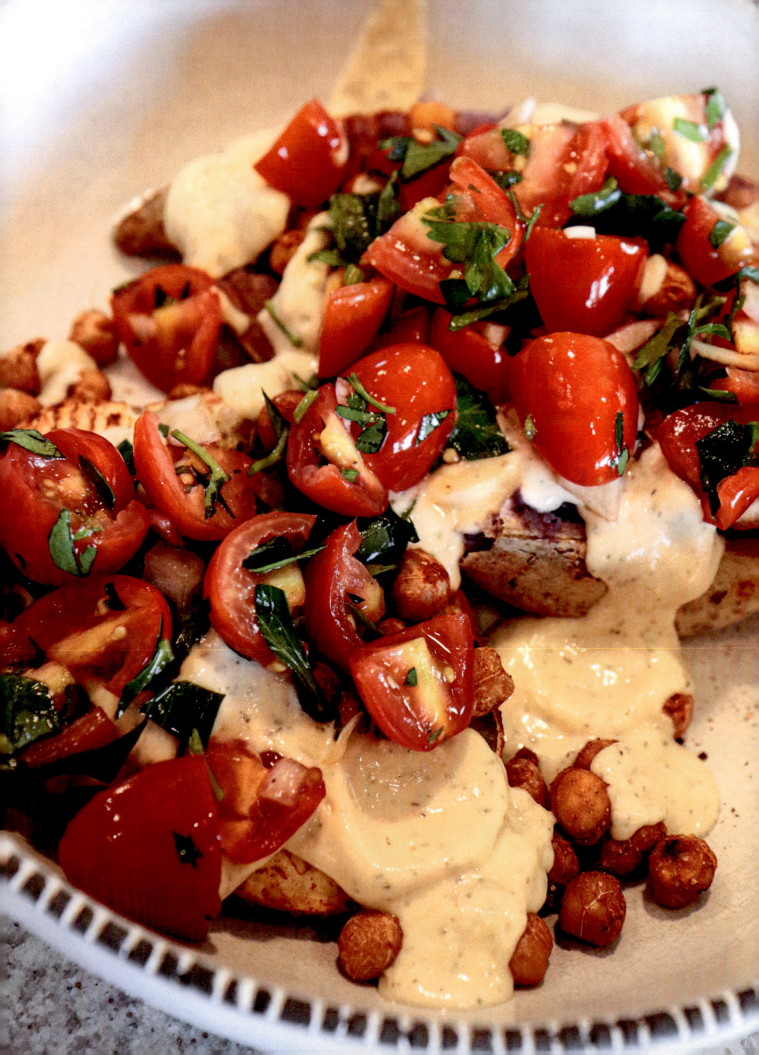

SUPPERS

LOADED SWEET POTATOES

This starchy meal is one of the best ways to enjoy sweet potatoes! The Garlic Herb Sauce is so good, definitely make a double batch to enjoy with bowls, veggies, grains, or salads!

INGREDIENTS

Loaded Sweet Potatoes
- 1 15 oz. can chickpeas, drained and rinsed
- 1 lemon, juiced
- 1 teaspoon ground cumin
- 1 teaspoon ground coriander
- 1 teaspoon ground cinnamon
- 1 teaspoon smoked paprika
- 4 large sweet potatoes, halved

Garlic Herb Sauce
- 1 15 oz. can chickpeas, drained and rinsed
- 1 tablespoon tahini (optional)
- 1 tablespoon lemon juice
- 5 garlic cloves, minced
- 1 1/4 cups soy milk
- 1 teaspoon dried dill (or 2 teaspoons fresh dill)

METHOD

Preheat the oven to 400°F.

In a mixing bowl, add all of the ingredients for the loaded potatoes except for the sweet potatoes. Mix together to evenly coat the chickpeas.

Spread the chickpea mixture onto a parchment-lined baking sheet along with the sweet potatoes face down. Place in the oven and bake for about 30 minutes or until the potatoes are tender.

Meanwhile, prepare the Garlic Herb Sauce by adding all the ingredients except the dill to a high-speed blender. Blend until smooth. Then add the dill and pulse quickly to combine. Set aside.

To assemble start with the sweet potatoes, then the chickpea mixture, and finally pour the sauce on top!

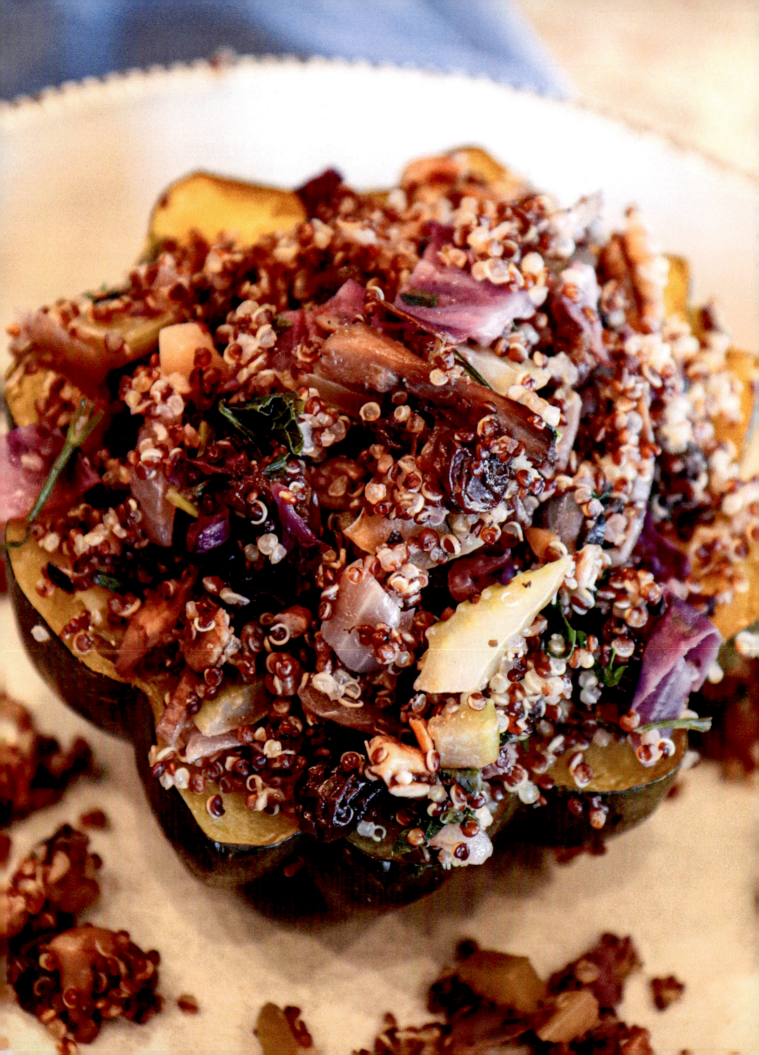

SUPPERS

STUFFED ACORN SQUASH

This recipe is an amazing way to impress your guests. While this dish might look super fancy, it is actually very simple to prepare! We love to make this one in the fall and winter when acorn squash are in season.

INGREDIENTS

- 2 acorn squash
- 3 ribs celery, diced
- 1 yellow onion, diced
- 4-6 mushrooms, chopped
- 1/2 cup red cabbage, chopped
- 1 apple, cored and diced
- 4 garlic cloves, minced
- black pepper, to taste
- 1/2 cup dried cranberries
- 1/2 cup pecans (optional)
- 1/2 bunch fresh parsley, chopped
- 3 cups cooked quinoa

METHOD

Preheat the oven to 375°F.

Cut the squash in half and remove the seeds. Place the squash into a glass baking dish cut side down. Add a little water, about 1/2 cup, to the bottom of the dish to keep from drying out while roasting. Cover with foil and roast for 40 minutes.

While the squash is baking, sauté the celery, onion, and mushrooms in a saucepan, adding a splash of veggie broth as needed to keep from sticking.

Once tender, add the cabbage, apple, garlic, and black pepper and sauté for another minute. Next, add the cranberries, pecans, and parsley. Sauté for a few more minutes to cook the flavors together and remove from heat.

In a large mixing bowl, add the quinoa and the sautéd mixture to make the filling. Stir well to combine.

Finally, stuff an acorn squash with the filling. Serve immediately or place in the oven for 10-15 minutes to caramelize the top.

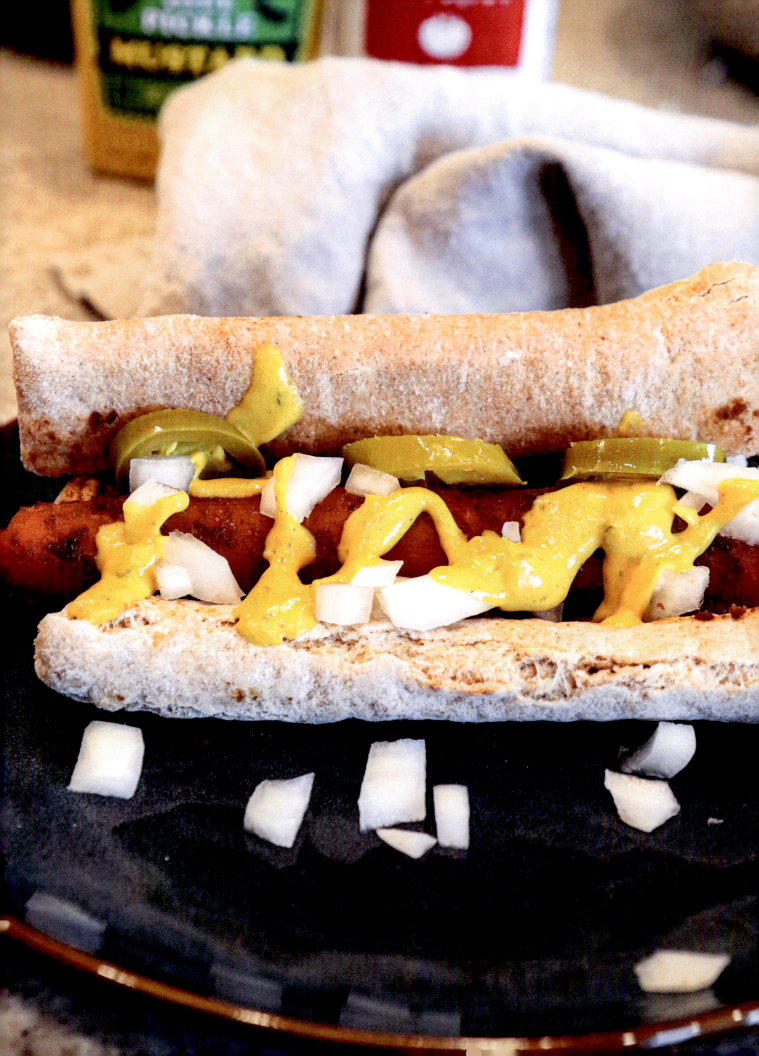

SUPPERS

CARROT DOGS

You haven't truly enjoyed a healthy hot dog until you've had a carrot dog! This marinade gives the carrots the most amazing flavor, while the simple cooking technique yields the perfect texture! Try making these at your next BBQ or picnic...they will be a hit!

INGREDIENTS

- 4-6 large carrots
- 1/4 cup veggie broth (or water)
- 2 tablespoons soy sauce (optional, but recommended)
- 3 tablespoons apple cider vinegar
- 2 teaspoons mustard
- 1/4 teaspoon allspice
- 1/4 teaspoon nutmeg
- 1/4 teaspoon smoked paprika
- 1/4 teaspoon cayenne pepper
- 1 teaspoon onion powder
- 1 teaspoon garlic powder
- a few drops of liquid smoke

METHOD

Cut the carrots at both ends to make them "hot-dog" length. If you wish, you can use a peeler to shape the carrots into a hot dog.

Steam the carrots 15-20 minutes until just fork tender, but don't overdo it. Submerge in an ice bath to cool.

Add the remaining ingredients to a mixing bowl and whisk to combine. Pour into a zipper bag.

Add the carrots to the bag and remove as much air as possible. Place the bag in the refrigerator to marinate for at least 12 hours or overnight.

To cook the carrot dogs, place them in a pan with the leftover marinade. Cook over medium heat until the liquid has simmered off, leaving the thick marinade coating the carrots.

Serve on a bun or bread with ketchup, mustard, onions, and any of your favorite toppings!

Note: Make a chili dog by topping with your favorite chili recipe! Enjoy all the nostalgic flavors by enjoying these dogs with the Baked Beans on page 75!

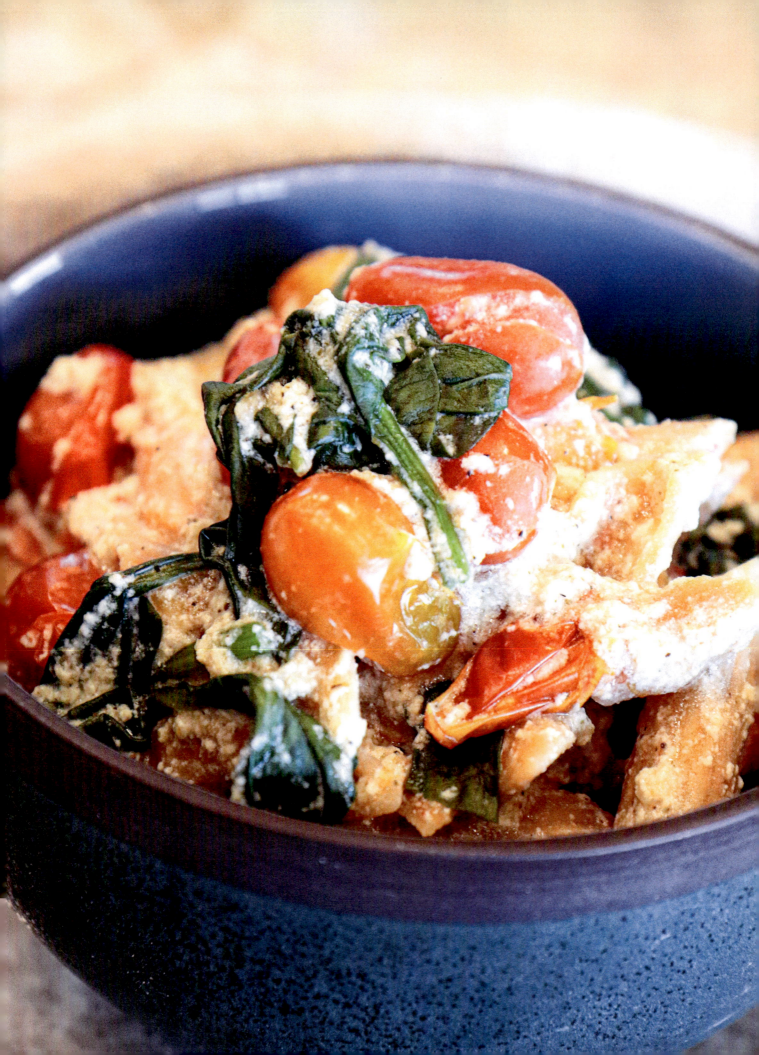

SUPPERS

TIKTOK FETA PASTA

We created this Instant Pot pasta because of a popular TikTok recipe using a block of feta, cherry tomatoes, and LOTS of oil. Luckily our version is plant-based, sos-free, and faster to whip up! Throw this one in the instant pot, no chopping needed!

INGREDIENTS

- 1   8 oz. box penne pasta
- 2   pints cherry tomatoes
- 2 1/2 cups water

- 2   teaspoons onion powder
- 1   tablespoon minced garlic
- 2   tablespoons apple cider vinegar
- 1   tablespoon Italian seasoning
- 1   14-16 oz. block firm tofu
- 1/2 cup water
- 1/4 cup nutritional yeast

- 1   5 oz. bag fresh baby spinach

METHOD

Add the pasta, cherry tomatoes, and 2 1/2 cups water to a pressure cooker.

To make the feta, add the remaining ingredients except for the spinach to a high-speed blender and blend until smooth.

Carefully pour the feta into the pressure cooker on top of the other ingredients. DO NOT STIR! Set to high pressure for 4 minutes, then manually release the pressure.

Finally, add the fresh spinach to the pressure cooker. Mix until the spinach is wilted.

Enjoy!

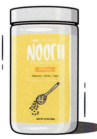

Our Well Your World Nooch is the tastiest non-fortified, nutritional yeast!

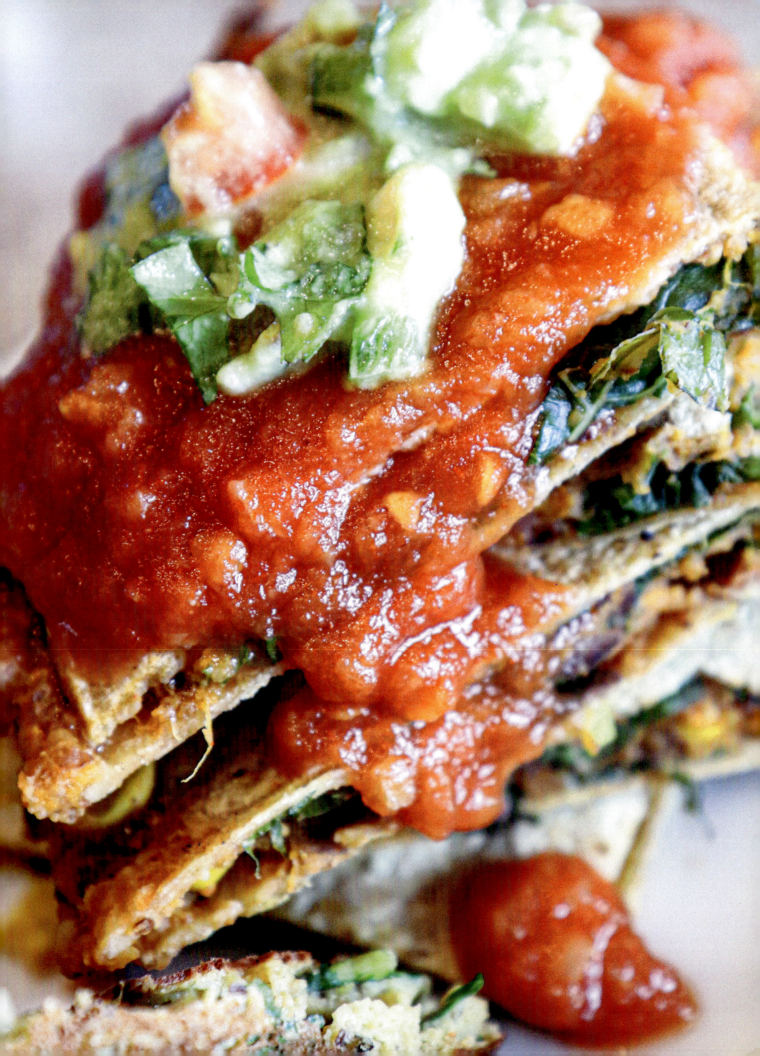

SUPPERS

QUESADILLAS

These quesadillas are packed full of starches and flavor! We love that these quesadillas leave you feeling full and satisfied without feeling weighed down. Enjoy topped with fresh guacamole and salsa.

INGREDIENTS

- 1 15 oz. can pinto beans, drained and rinsed
- 1 15 oz. can black beans, drained and rinsed
- 1 sweet potato, cooked
- 1/2 cup corn
- 3-5 garlic cloves, minced
- 1/2 teaspoon dried oregano
- 1-2 teaspoons chili powder (optional)
- 3-4 leaves kale, de-stemmed and chopped
- 2-4 tortillas

METHOD

Add the pinto and black beans to a large mixing bowl. Mash well with a potato masher or a fork. Add the remaining ingredients except for the tortillas and mix well to create the filling.

To prepare the quesadillas, preheat a non-stick skillet or electric griddle to 350°F. Place a tortilla down onto the cooking surface, spoon some of the filling onto the middle and spread evenly. Allow to cook for 5-10 minutes.

Next, add the top tortilla and flip to cook the other side. Cook for an additional 5 minutes.

To serve, cut the quesadilla into quarters. Top with pico de gallo, hot sauce, salsa, or diced avocado!

Note: To cook in a panini press, spoon the filling onto a tortilla and spread evenly. Add the top tortilla and press the panini press closed. Cook for 10-15 minutes.

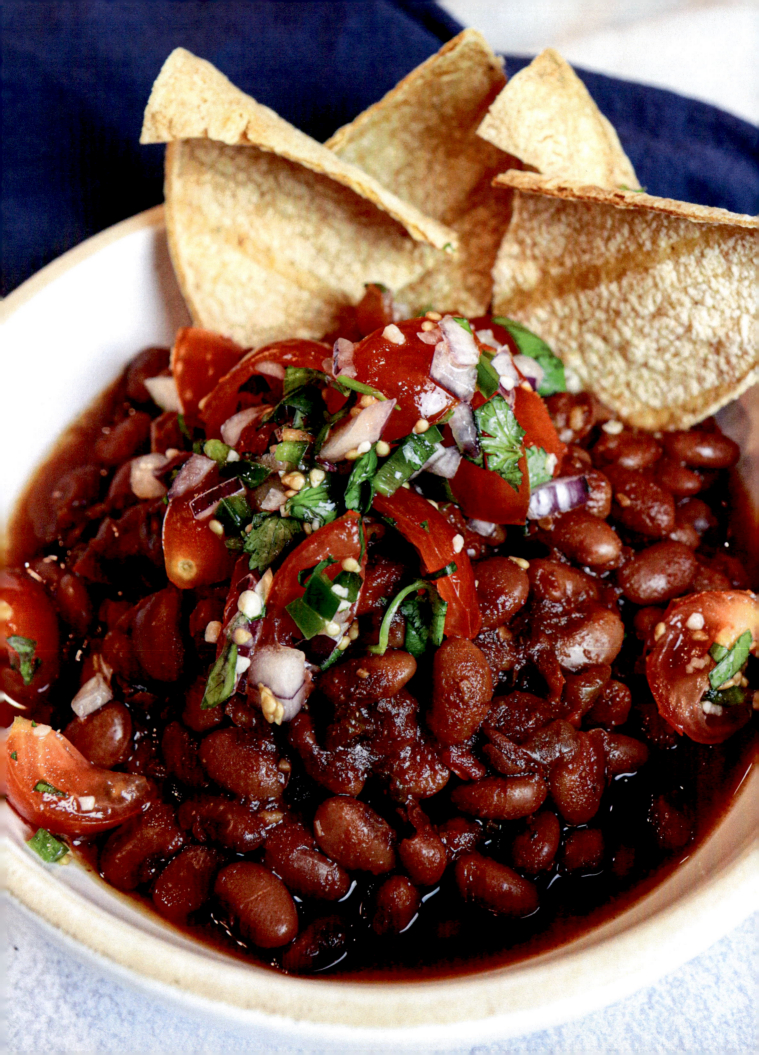

SUPPERS

MEXICAN CHARRO BEANS

This recipe is one Dillon used to eat every single day for lunch while working on rooftops installing solar panels before he started Well Your World. Make a batch to enjoy all week long just like Dillon did (and still does). Don't forget a monster batch of Pico too!

INGREDIENTS

- 1 yellow onion, diced
- 1 red bell pepper, diced
- 2 jalapeños, seeded and diced
- 1/4 cup chili powder
- 2 teaspoons ground cumin
- 1 tablespoon dried oregano
- 1 tablespoon minced garlic
- 3 bay leaves
- 1 15oz. can tomato sauce
- 2 cups veggie broth
- 2 lbs dry pinto beans
- water, to fill line (about 5 cups)

- pico de gallo, to serve
- tortilla chips, to serve

METHOD

Add all of the ingredients to a 6-quart Instant Pot or pressure cooker. Set to high pressure for 45 minutes with a 15 minute natural release for al dente beans. Set to high pressure for 1 hour with a 15 minute natural release for softer beans.

Top with fresh pico and enjoy with homemade tortilla chips to really take it to the next level. Enjoy!

Note: Using boiling water will allow your pressure cooker to heat up more quickly.

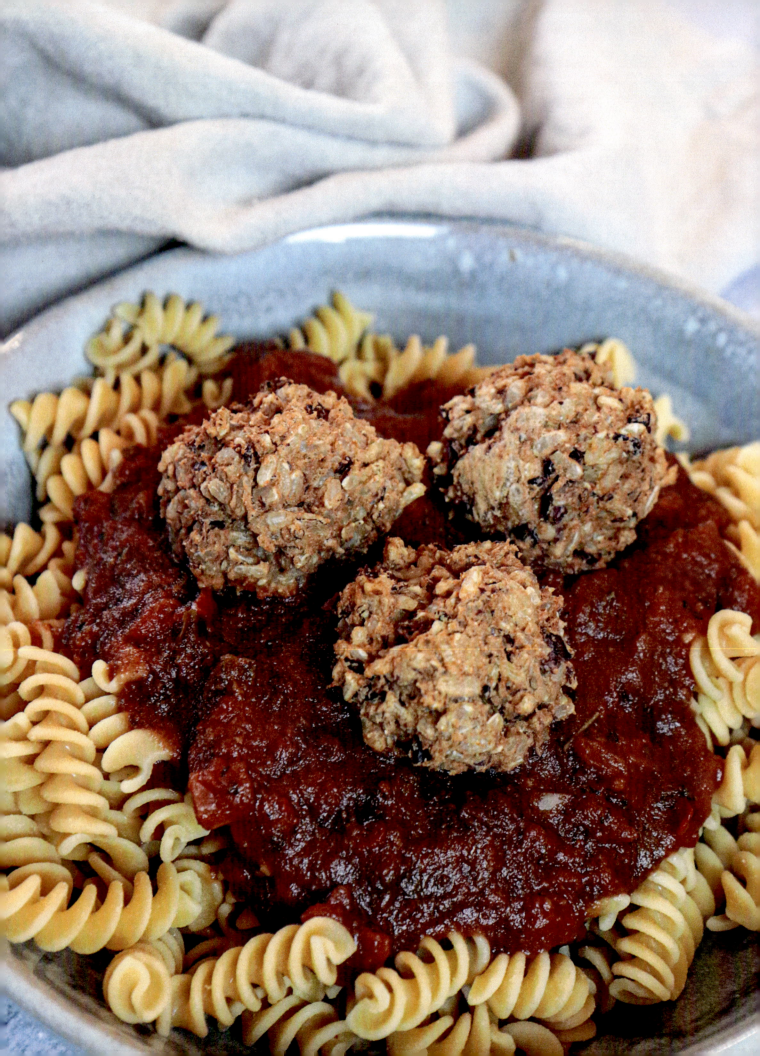

SUPPERS

3-INGREDIENT STARCHBALLS

Easily take your pasta dishes up a notch with these Starchballs! These are also great for dipping and enjoying on their own too.

INGREDIENTS

- 1   15 oz. can kidney beans, drained and rinsed
- 1   10 oz. bag frozen rice
- 2   tablespoons chickpea flour
- 1   tablespoon WYW Voodoo or Cajun seasoning blend
- 1   teaspoon WYW Stardust or salt substitute

METHOD

Preheat the oven to 400°F.

Add everything to a large mixing bowl and mash with a potato masher or just use your hands!

Roll the mixture into 1" balls and lay on a parchment lined baking sheet. Bake for about 20 minutes.

Serve them over your favorite pasta dish or dip them in your favorite sauce!

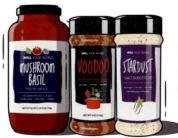

Our pasta sauces and seasonings can help make this meal super fast!

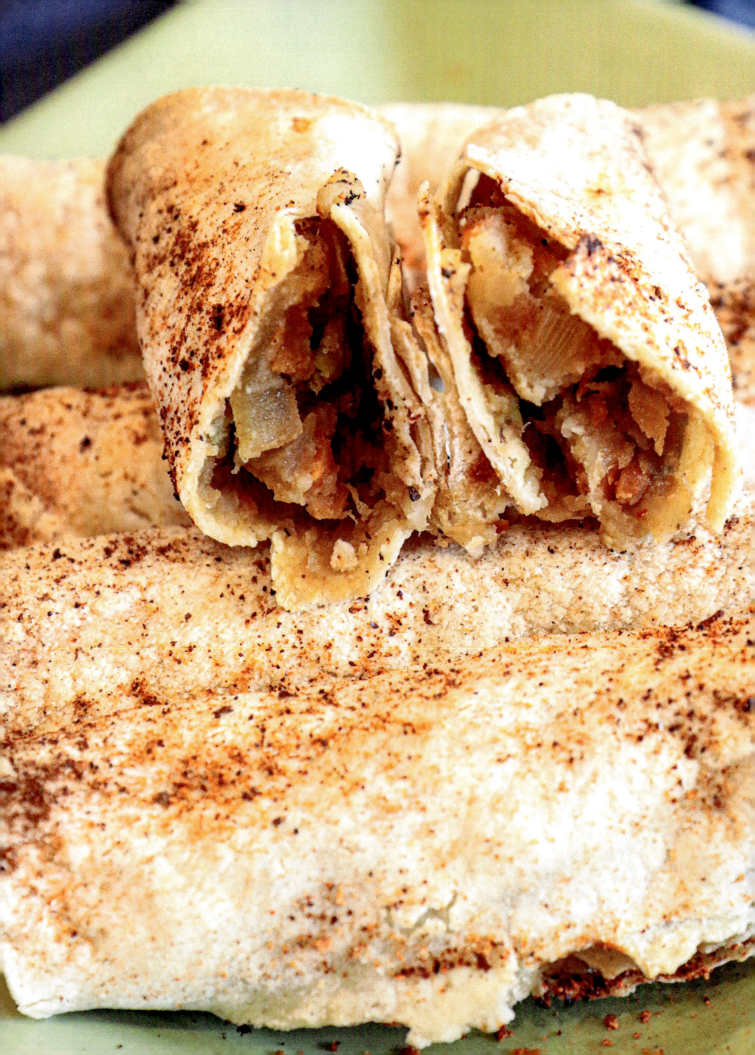

SUPPERS

SAMOSA TAQUITOS

This recipe has the classic Indian flavors of a samosa rolled into a tortilla making it so simple to throw together. Dip in WYW Indian Everything Sauce!

INGREDIENTS

- 2 medium russet potatoes, peeled & chopped
- 2 tablespoons soy milk
- 1 10-12 oz. bag frozen peas and carrots mix
- 1 small yellow onion, diced
- 3 garlic cloves, minced
- 1 teaspoon curry powder
- 1 teaspoon onion powder
- 1 teaspoon ground cumin
- 1/4 teaspoon ground turmeric
- 1 teaspoon smoked paprika
- 1/2 teaspoon crushed red pepper (optional)
- black pepper, to taste

- corn tortillas
- lime/lemon juice
- WYW Chili Lime

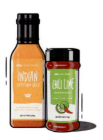

METHOD

Preheat the oven to 400°F.

Add the chopped potatoes to a small saucepan and cover with water. Boil for about 7 minutes until tender then strain out the water. Add the potatoes to a mixing bowl along with the soy milk and mash until mostly smooth.

Next, add the peas & carrots, onion, garlic, and all of the spices to a saucepan over medium high heat and sauté for 5-7 minutes, adding some water or veggie broth as needed to keep from sticking. Cook until the carrots are tender.

Add the sauté mixture to the mashed potatoes and stir well to combine into a thick filling.

To assemble, warm the tortillas so they do not split apart by microwaving in a towel for 20-30 seconds. Add a couple tablespoons of filling, roll them up, then place on a parchment-lined baking sheet seam side down.

Squeeze on some lemon or lime juice over top and sprinkle on some WYW Chili Lime. This step is optional but adds a nice touch!

Bake for 17 mins or until your desired crispiness. Dip in WYW Indian Sauce and enjoy!

Note: Using pre-cooked leftover potatoes in this recipe makes it even faster!

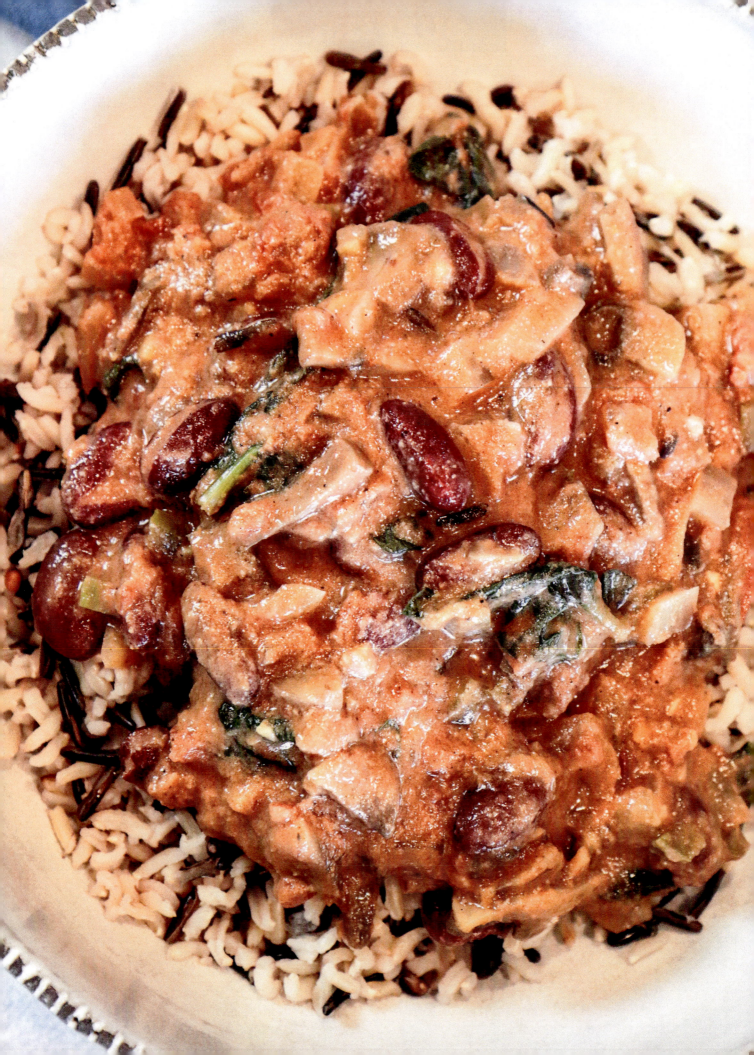

SUPPERS

MUSHROOM KIDNEY BEAN CURRY

This recipe really has it all...starches, grains, veggies, greens, and more! Plus it is so fast to make that it will have you eating in 20 minutes or less and can be prepared in so many different ways.

INGREDIENTS

Low Fat Coconut Milk
- 1 cup soy milk
- 1 1/2 tablespoons plain shredded coconut

Curry
- 1 yellow onion, diced
- 1/2 lb. mushrooms, sliced
- 1/2" fresh ginger, peeled and minced
- 3 garlic cloves, minced
- 1 jalapeño, diced small
- 1 tablespoon garam masala
- 2 teaspoons ground cumin
- 2 teaspoons ground coriander
- 1 15 oz. can diced tomatoes
- 1 15 oz. can kidney beans, drained and rinsed
- 1 teaspoon WYW Date Powder (optional)
- 2 cups fresh spinach
- 1/2 lime, juiced

METHOD

To make the Low Fat Coconut Milk, add the ingredients to a blender and blend until smooth. Set aside.

Add the onion, mushrooms, ginger, garlic, and jalapeño to a saucepan and sauté over medium-high heat for 3-5 minutes or until tender, adding a splash of water or veggie broth as needed to keep from sticking.

Add the garam masala, cumin, and coriander, and sauté for a couple more minutes, adding more liquid as needed.

Add the tomatoes, kidney beans, and date powder to the saucepan along with the Coconut Milk and bring to a simmer. Then add the spinach gradually and stir to wilt. Finally, add the lime juice, stir and enjoy!

We love this over any cooked starch like rice, quinoa, or potatoes.

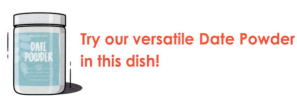

Try our versatile Date Powder in this dish!

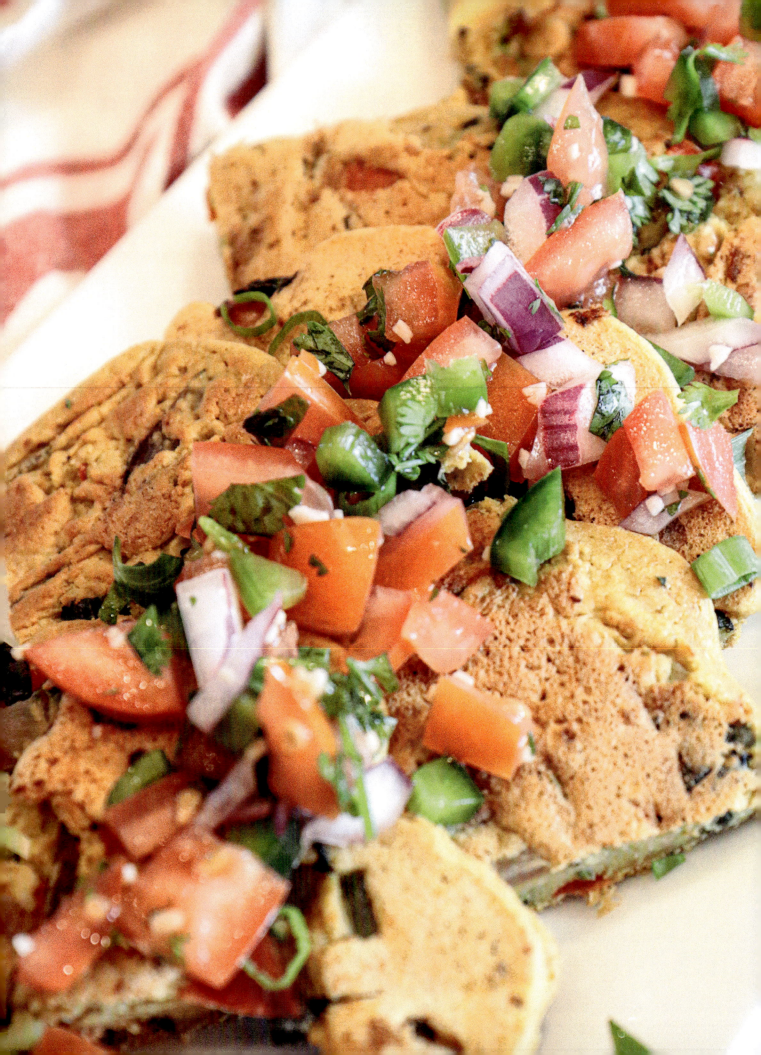

SUPPERS

CHICKPEA OMELET

Don't save this meal for only breakfast! This one is so quick to whip up and is a great way to use up any veggies you have on hand. It's delicious, starchy, and filling!

INGREDIENTS

Chickpea Batter
- 1 cup chickpea flour
- 1 teaspoon onion powder
- 1/2 teaspoon paprika
- 1 teaspoon garlic powder
- 1/4 teaspoon black pepper
- 1/4 teaspoon turmeric
- 1/4 teaspoon black salt (optional)
- 1 teaspoon baking powder
- 1/3 cup nutritional yeast
- 1 cup + 2 tablespoons soy milk

Omelet Veggies
- diced onion
- chopped mushrooms
- diced green pepper
- chopped zucchini
- diced bell pepper
- chopped spinach

Toppings
- salsa
- pico de gallo
- chopped cherry tomatoes
- sliced green onion

METHOD

Preheat a non-stick electric griddle to 350°F.

Add all of the dry Chickpea Batter ingredients to a large mixing bowl and whisk together. Then whisk in the soy milk.

Next, add as much of the veggies you would like to the batter, adding more soy milk if it becomes too thick. Stir well to combine.

This recipe will make two omelets, so pour about half the batter out onto the griddle. Feel free to lift and tilt the griddle to spread the batter around. You don't want your omelet to be too thick or it will not cook through.

After a couple minutes, use a plastic/rubber spatula to carefully flip your omelet then press down a bit to make good contact with the griddle.

Cook for 5-10 minutes, just until you reach your desired level of doneness. Top with your favorite items from the toppings list and enjoy!

Note: This works best on a simple, non-stick griddle like the one pictured below!

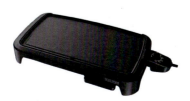

THANK YOU!

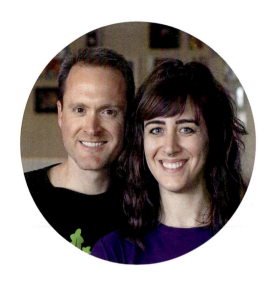

A sincere thank you for your support!
♡ Dillon & Reebs ♡

Thank you so much for ALL you do to support us, whether it's purchasing this book, watching our YouTube videos, liking an Instagram post, or ordering our products.

We are so grateful to have a like-minded community of awesome people who appreciate all of the hard work we put into teaching you and others how simple it is to eat healthy!

If you have any questions or comments, you can always email us at: hello@wellyourworld.com

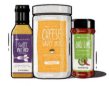

▶ youtube.com/wellyourworld

f facebook.com/groups/wellyourworld

◉ @wellyourworld

✉ hello@wellyourworld.com

WELL YOUR WEEKEND!

If you love delicious, plant-based, SOS-free recipes like the ones in this cookbook, you'll LOVE our live interactive cooking show, Well Your Weekend. We go live twice a month and feature 3-4 new recipes every show. Members get access to all past replays and recipe PDF's!

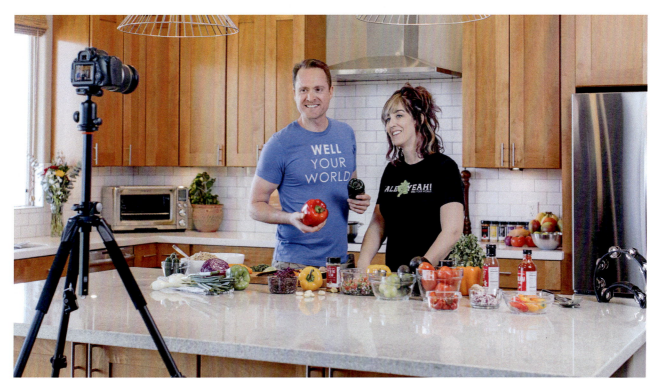

- 2 ENTERTAINING LIVE COOKING SHOWS PER MONTH
- 10% MEMBERS-ONLY DISCOUNT ON ALL WYW PRODUCTS
- BRAND NEW PLANT-BASED, OIL-FREE RECIPES EVERY SHOW
- ACCESS TO 125+ REPLAY VIDEOS & 400+ RECIPE DOWNLOADS
- COMMUNITY INTERACTION WITH OTHERS WHO EAT LIKE YOU!
- $15/MONTH, NO COMMITMENT, CANCEL ANYTIME

SIGN UP NOW!

WELLYOURWORLD.COM/COOKING SHOW

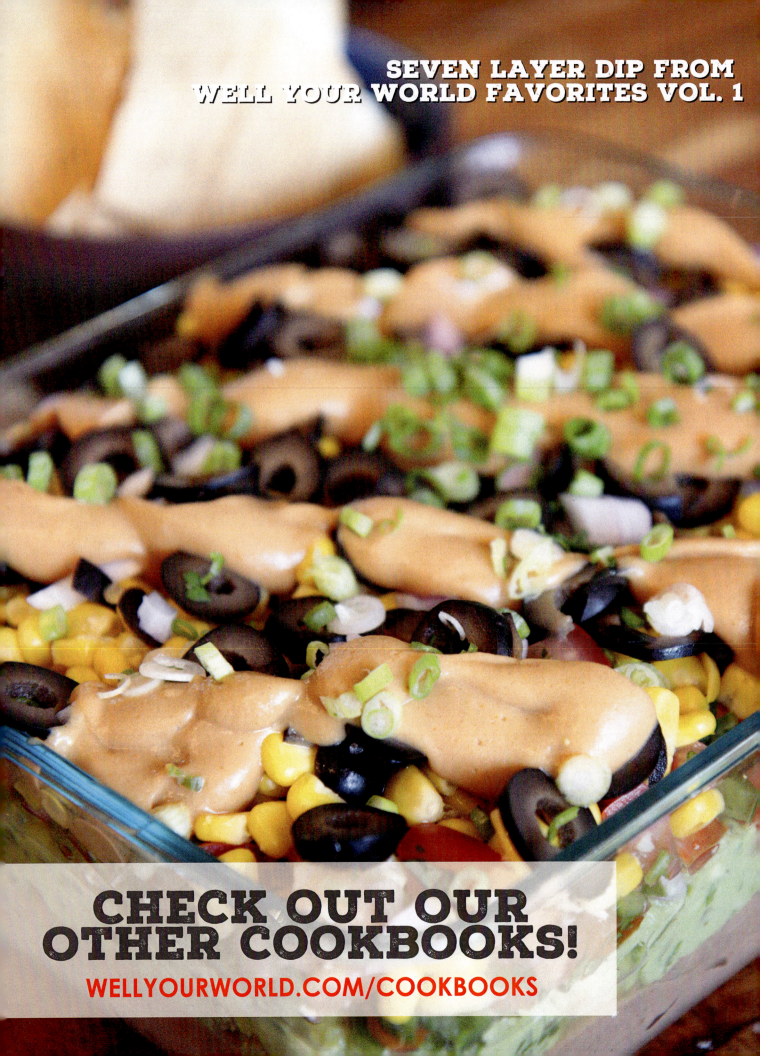

PURCHASE OUR OTHER COOKBOOKS!

Looking for more inspiration in the kitchen? Check out our three cookbooks, all with full color photos for each recipe, available in digital or hardcopy format. Packed with simple, no-fuss ingredients and methods, our cookbooks will help you simplify your healthy diet!

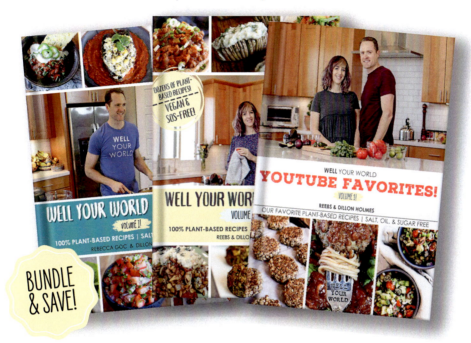

ALL OF OUR COOKBOOKS HAVE:

- BEAUTIFUL FULL PAGE PHOTOS FOR EVERY RECIPE
- EASY TO FIND INGREDIENTS
- DOZENS OF WHOLE FOOD PLANT-BASED AND SALT, OIL, AND SUGAR FREE RECIPES
- EASY TO FOLLOW INSTRUCTIONS FOR BEGINNERS AND VETERANS ALIKE
- PAPERBACK AND DIGITAL FORMATS AVAILABLE
- TIPS AND TRICKS FOR A PLANT-BASED LIFESTYLE
- FREE SHIPPING TO THE USA

↪ **WELLYOURWORLD.COM/COOKBOOKS**

SIMPLIFY YOUR DIET WITH WELL YOUR WORLD PRODUCTS!

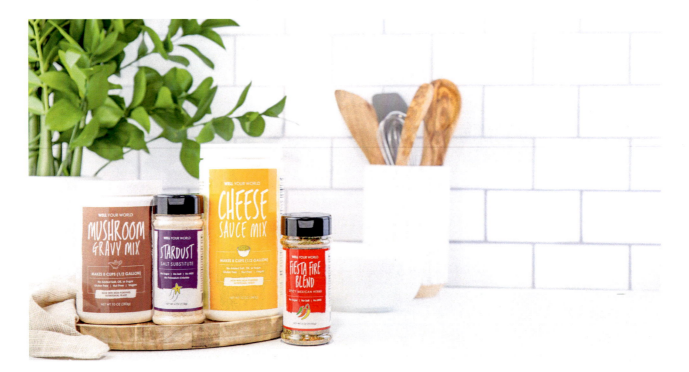

Now you can simplify your healthy diet without sacrificing time or flavor with our Well Your World lineup of whole food products.

Our time-saving pantry items make it easy to stay on track thanks to staples like our Cheese Sauce Mix, spice blends, and simmer sauces.

Check out our complete line of sauces, spices, mixes, dressings and more!

SHOP NOW!

↳ **WELLYOURWORLD.COM**

FREE USA SHIPPING ON ALL ORDERS $50 OR MORE!